Trends in Andrology and Sexual Medicine

Series editors
Emmanuele A. Jannini
Chair of Endocrinology and Sexology (Endosex)
Department of Systems Medicine
University of Rome Tor Vergata
Italy

Mario Maggi
Andrology Unit
University of Florence
Italy

Carlo Foresta
Department of Histology, Microbiology, and Medical Biotechnologies
Center for Male Gamete Cryopreservation
University of Padua
Italy

Andrea Lenzi
Department of Experimental Medicine
Sapienza University of Rome
Italy

This series will serve as a comprehensive and authoritative resource that presents state of the art knowledge and practice within the fields of Andrology and Sexual Medicine, covering basic science and clinical and psychological aspects. Each volume will focus on a specific topic relating to reproductive or sexual health, such as male and female sexual disorders (from erectile dysfunction to vaginismus, and from hypoactive desire to ejaculatory disturbances), diagnostic issues in infertility and sexual dysfunction, and current and emerging therapies (from assisted reproduction techniques to testosterone supplementation, and from PDE5i to SSRIs for premature ejaculation). In addition, selected new topics not previously covered in a single monograph will be addressed, examples including male osteoporosis and the approach of traditional Chinese medicine to sexual medicine. Against the background of rapid progress in Andrology and Sexual Medicine, the series will meet the need of readers for detailed updates on new discoveries in physiology and pathophysiology and in the therapy of human sexual and reproductive disorders.

More information about this series at http://www.springer.com/series/13846

Giancarlo Balercia • Loredana Gandini
Andrea Lenzi • Francesco Lombardo
Editors

Antioxidants in Andrology

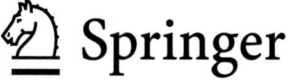 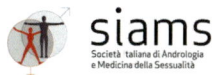

Editors

Giancarlo Balercia
Endocrinology Department
Polytechnic University of Marche
Ancona
Italy

Loredana Gandini†
Department of Experimental Medicine
Section of Medical Pathophysiology
Sapienza University of Rome
Rome
Italy

Andrea Lenzi
Department of Experimental Medicine
Section of Medical Pathophysiology
Sapienza University of Rome
Rome
Italy

Francesco Lombardo
Department of Experimental Medicine
Section of Medical Pathophysiology
Sapienza University of Rome
Rome
Italy

ISSN 2367-0088   ISSN 2367-0096   (electronic)
Trends in Andrology and Sexual Medicine
ISBN 978-3-319-41747-9   ISBN 978-3-319-41749-3   (eBook)
DOI 10.1007/978-3-319-41749-3

Library of Congress Control Number: 2016960198

Printed on acid-free paper

This Springer imprint is published by Springer Nature
The registered company is Springer International Publishing AG
The registered company address is Gewerbestrasse 11, 6330 Cham, Switzerland

Dedication

Professor Loredana Gandini passed away because a sudden and dramatic disease on October 5, 2016, at the Umberto I General Hospital, in the same Sapienza University of Rome where she was an esteemed lecturer. Born in 1953 in the North of Italy, she obtained in 1980 the Degree in Biological Sciences and, four years later, the Degree of Specialist in General Pathology. At the end of her too short life, she was Full Professor of Clinical Pathology (since 2008) in the Sapienza University of Rome, Director of the Master in Andrology and Seminology, Director of the Complex Unit "Endocrine Diagnostics and Sperm Bank". Professor Gandini wrote a number of very well-cited full papers on international journals and more than 100 textbooks, manuals, book chapters, and monographs. She served as President of the Italian Society of Embryology, Reproduction and Research; Member of the Board of Directors of the Italian Society of Andrology and Sexual Medicine, and President of the Italian Society of Reproductive Pathophysiology.

Loredana Gandini was very active in the field of Endocrinology-Andrology, Reproductive Pathophysiology, and Immunology of Reproduction. She performed a constant and well-recognized effort to study, with modern techniques, the sperm physiology and male infertility. Most of the methods she developed have been transferred into the clinical setting.

She had always demonstrated her scientific and intellectual honesty both as Teacher and Scientist that did make her very well recognized in the field of Reproductive Medicine, Endocrinology and Embryology, and Andrology but also she had a wonderful smile that could light up a room.

This book is dedicated to Lori, as we affectionately called her, outstanding figure of scientist and our friend of a lifetime.

Contents

Free Radicals in Andrology

Ashok Agarwal and Ahmad Majzoub

1.1   Introduction

Infertility is a condition associated with major medical and social preoccupation. A male etiology is responsible for nearly half the cases of infertility [1] and is caused by alterations in sperm concentration, motility, and/or morphology [2]. Recent advances in the field of infertility have greatly influenced our understanding of the different circumstances attributing to male factor infertility. While environmental, physiological, and genetic influences were recognized, at the molecular level, oxidative stress (OS) resulting from the imbalance between oxidants and reductants appears to be a common denominator impairing sperm function and delaying pregnancy.

Reactive oxygen species (ROS) are highly reactive oxidizing agents that can, at supraphysiological levels, have a potential toxic effect on sperm quality and function [3]. Like other free radicals, ROS contain unpaired electrons triggering a tendency for strong reactivity with other compounds. Moreover, they typically incite a chain reaction exposing a *vicious circle* type of activity. Under normal physiological circumstances, ROS are products of natural oxygen metabolism acting as vital signaling molecules. However, excessive levels of ROS can be

A. Agarwal, PhD, HCLD (✉)
American Center for Reproductive Medicine, Department of Urology, Cleveland Clinic, Cleveland, OH 44195, USA

Lerner College of Medicine, Andrology Center and American Center for Reproductive Medicine, 10681 Carnegie Avenue, Desk X11, Cleveland, OH 44195, USA
e-mail: agarwaa@ccf.org; http://www.ClevelandClinic.Org/ReproductiveResearchCenter

A. Majzoub, MD
American Center for Reproductive Medicine, Department of Urology, Cleveland Clinic, Cleveland, OH 44195, USA

© Springer International Publishing Switzerland 2017
G. Balercia et al. (eds.), *Antioxidants in Andrology*, Trends in Andrology and Sexual Medicine, DOI 10.1007/978-3-319-41749-3_1

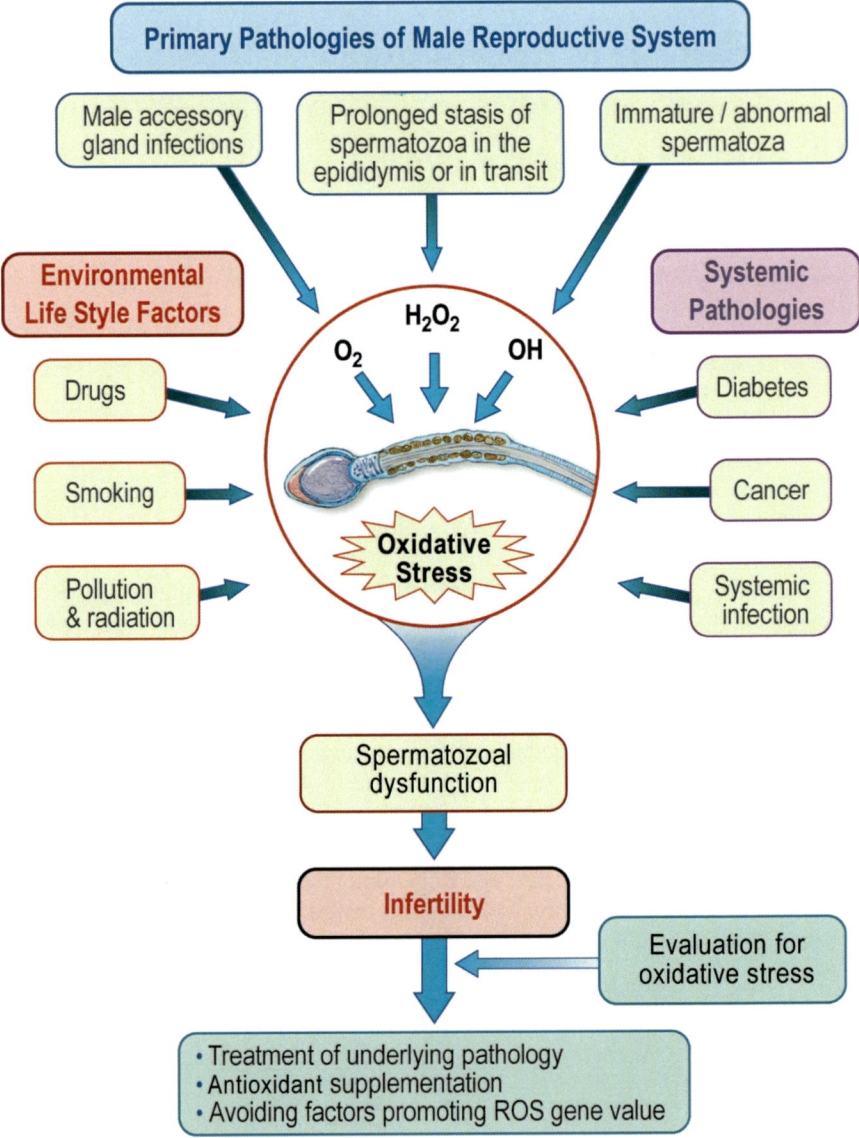

Fig. 1.1 Factors contributing to oxidative stress-induced male infertility (Copyright license provided)

produced secondary to a variety of environmental exposures and pathologic processes (Fig. 1.1) resulting in several disease entities such as neurodegenerative disease, vascular disease, cancer, and infertility. To minimize the hazardous effects of excessive ROS levels, a number of endogenous enzymatic and nonenzymatic antioxidants exist scavenging or neutralizing excess ROS.

Like all other living cells, spermatozoa require oxygen for survival. However, excessive exposure to oxygen metabolites can alter normal sperm function and vitality [3, 4]. Several reports have confirmed the presence of high ROS levels in the semen of 25–40 % of infertile men [5, 6]. Negative correlations were detected between ROS levels and normal sperm morphology as well as with measures of sperm DNA fragmentation [7, 8]. Spermatozoa are predominantly vulnerable to the damage caused by excessive ROS because their plasma membranes contain extraordinary large amounts of polyunsaturated fatty acids (PUFA) [9], and their cytoplasm contains very low concentrations of scavenging enzymes [10]. These intracellular antioxidant enzymes cannot protect the plasma membrane that surrounds the acrosome and the tail, forcing spermatozoa to depend on the protection provided by the seminal plasma.

This review discusses the mechanisms by which ROS develop in semen and their role in the pathophysiology of male infertility. Topics include the clinical implications of high levels of seminal ROS, the different methods available for ROS detection, and a treatment strategy for infertile men in whom OS is found to be influential.

1.2   ROS Generation

The family of ROS includes oxygen-centered radicals such as the superoxide anion radical ($\cdot O_2^-$), hydroxyl radical (OH$\cdot$), and nitric oxide radical (NO$\cdot$), in addition to non-radical derivatives, such as hydrogen peroxide (H_2O_2), peroxynitrite anion (ONOO$^-$), and hypochlorous acid (HOCL) [11].

A variety of semen components, including sperm with abnormal morphology, germ cells, and leukocytes, are capable of generating ROS. Seminal leukocytes and morphologically abnormal spermatozoa are the main sources of ROS in human ejaculates [12].

1.2.1   Reactive Oxygen Species Production by Spermatozoa

Human spermatozoa can produce ROS in one of two ways: (1) through the nicotinamide adenine dinucleotide phosphate (NADPH) oxidase system at the level of the sperm plasma membrane and (2) through the NADH-dependent oxidoreductase (diphorase) system at the level of mitochondria [13]. Damaged spermatozoa are an established source of excessive ROS production [14]. The increase in ROS generation is thought to result from excess residual cytoplasm (cytoplasmic droplets) typically present in abnormal spermatozoa. During spermatogenesis, defects in cytoplasmic extrusion result in the development of immature sperm containing a surplus of residual cytoplasm [15]. ROS generation has been positively correlated with the extent of residual cytoplasmic retention. This observation is thought to be mediated by the concurrent increase in the enzyme glucose-6-phosphate-dehydrogenase (G6PD) activity seen in abnormal spermatozoa. G6PD stimulates glucose influx through the hexose monophosphate shunt raising the intracellular availability of NADPH, a major source of electrons for spermatozoa used to fuel the generation of ROS [16].

Creatine kinase (CK), a biochemical marker of cytoplasmic space, has been correlated with the degree of oxidative damage in human sperm. Alani and El Yaseen [17] have found a significant positive correlation between CK activity and malondialdehyde (MDA) formation in sperm fractions from infertile men. Hallak et al. demonstrated an inverse relationship between CK levels and sperm morphological forms suggesting that CK levels can be used to reliably predict sperm quality and fertilizing potential in men with infertility [18].

Since spermatozoa are rich in mitochondria in order to supply the necessary energy needed for motility, the major source of ROS in spermatozoa in infertile men originates from the mitochondria. Mitochondrial dysfunction has been associated with increased ROS production [19], which results in more damage to the mitochondrial membrane and consequently fuels more ROS production.

Superoxide is the primary ROS generated in human spermatozoa [20]. This one-electron molecule is capable of reacting with itself in a dismutation reaction to generate H_2O_2 and $O_2\cdot$. In the presence of transition metals such as iron and copper, it can interact to generate $OH\cdot$ through the Haber-Weiss reaction ($\cdot O_2^- + H_2O_2 \rightarrow OH\cdot + OH + O_2$). Alternatively, $OH\cdot$ can be produced from H_2O_2 through the Fenton reaction, which requires ferrous ions as reducing agents ($H_2O_2 + Fe^{2+} \rightarrow Fe^{3+} + OH\cdot + OH$). The $OH\cdot$ is thought to be the most hazardous ROS initiating the lipid peroxidation (LPO) cascade and causing loss of sperm functions [21].

1.2.2   ROS Production by Leukocytes

Leukocytospermia has been largely considered as a major cause of male infertility [22]. Peroxidase-positive leukocytes include polymorphonuclear leukocytes and macrophages which represent 50 % and 30 % of all seminal leukocytes, respectively [23], while T lymphocytes constitute the remaining 10 % of seminal leukocytes [23]. They are mainly released with prostatic and seminal vesicle secretions and are capable of producing large amounts of ROS in response to infection or inflammation [22]. Once activated, the leukocytes' myeloperoxidase system is stimulated leading to an oxidative burst that provides the early defense system against microbes in cases of infection.

Sperm damage from leukocyte-produced ROS can occur after removal of seminal plasma during preparations performed for assisted reproduction or when leukocytospermia exists. A recent study by Lobascio et al. [12] demonstrated the presence of a positive correlation between the number of seminal leukocytes and ROS levels ($p < 0.001$; $n = 125$). Moreover, they confirmed the negative consequence of such a relationship through finding significant negative correlations with sperm concentration ($p = 0.01$) and motility ($p = 0.02$) and a positive correlation with sperm DNA fragmentation (SDF) ($p = 0.08$) [12]. Mupfiga et al. investigated semen samples from 60 infertile patients and found higher ROS production and caspase activity, a marker of apoptosis, in samples containing a higher number of leukocytes [24]. Saleh et al. [25] compared semen samples from 48 infertile men with those from healthy volunteers. To objectively assess leukocyte-ROS production, samples from patients with no evidence of leukocytospermia ($n = 32$) were further incubated with blood neutrophils. In comparison with samples from healthy volunteers and non-leukoctospermic infertile men, significantly higher levels of ROS were detected in samples from leukocytospermic infertile men or after incubation with blood neutrophils. Furthermore, the authors demonstrated a significant decrease in sperm motility and increase in sperm DNA damage in leukocytospermic samples [25].

Sperm damage from leukocyte-derived ROS may happen even at leukocyte concentrations below the World Health Organization's cutoff value for leukocytospermia, that is, greater than 1×10^6 peroxidase-positive leukocytes/mL of semen [26]. In a comparative study, Agarwal et al. divided semen samples from 472 infertile men into three groups: group 1, no seminal leukocytes; group 2, low-level leukocytospermia (0.1–1.0×10^6 WBC/mL); and group 3, frank leukocytospermia ($>1.0 \times 10^6$ WBC/mL). Results revealed significantly higher levels of ROS and sperm DNA fragmentation in group 2 samples (ROS, 1839.65 ± 2173.57 RLU/s; DNA damage, 26.47 ± 19.64 %) compared with group 1 samples (ROS, 1101.09 ± 5557.54 RLU/s; DNA damage, 19.89 ± 17.31 %) (ROS, $p = 0.002$; DNA damage, $p = 0.047$), without significant differences detected between groups 2 and 3. Finally, seminal leukocytes may induce ROS production by human spermatozoa through a mechanism that is not clearly understood [25].

1.3   ROS and Sperm Physiology

At optimal levels, ROS exhibit favorable effects that can potentiate sperm fertilizing capabilities. Fertilization is key to normal conception. It requires ideal oocyte and sperm conditions to successfully occur. After spermiation, the spermatozoa must mature within the male genital tract and undergo capacitation and acrosome reaction during their passage in the female tract. Such steps are necessary before penetrating the zona pellucida of the ova and fusing with the female pronucleus. Studies have shown that the incubation of spermatozoa with H_2O_2 stimulates sperm capacitation, hyperactivation, acrosome reaction, and oocyte fusion [27–29].

Other ROS, such as $\cdot O_2^-$ and NO, have also been shown to promote sperm capacitation and acrosome reaction [30]. Capacitation usually starts after an increase in intracellular calcium, followed by an increase in cyclic adenosine monophosphate (cAMP), activation of protein kinase A, and consequent tyrosine kinase activation resulting in the development of a highly vigorous form of motility known as hyperactivation. Studies have shown that H_2O_2 is specifically involved in capacitation through its ability to increase cAMP levels [31]. Upon approaching the oocyte, a sudden influx of extracellular calcium into the acrosomal region occurs due to the influence of progesterone. This causes the spermatozoa to become highly sensitized and ready to undergo the acrosome reaction [28]. Sperm-oocyte fusion was found to be mediated by signaling events that occur in low concentrations of H_2O_2 [32]. Aitken et al. revealed that low levels of ROS augment the ability of spermatozoa to bind with the zona pellucida, an effect that was reversed by the addition of vitamin E [33].

1.4   Consequences of Excessive Generation of ROS

Almost every human ejaculate contains potential sources of ROS, namely, leukocytes, immature spermatozoa, and precursor germ cells. It is generally accepted that OS and the consequent loss of sperm function occur in every ejaculate, however, to a variable extent that depends on the nature, amount, and timing of ROS exposure. Excessive seminal ROS levels have been implicated in the pathophysiology of male infertility through their detrimental effects on the following:

1.4.1   ROS and Apoptosis

Apoptosis or programmed cell death is a noninflammatory response to tissue injury characterized by a series of biochemical changes leading to changes in cellular morphology and death. A stringently regulated apoptosis is essential for normal development of spermatozoa as well as the adjustment of the number of sperm cells that are produced [34]. On the other hand, a process termed "abortive apoptosis," occurring during spermatogenesis, has been associated with male infertility [35–38].

While apoptosis may be triggered by several intrinsic and extrinsic factors, ROS levels appear to be directly correlated with the extent of sperm cell death. Mostafa et al. demonstrated the presence of higher levels of ROS which correlated with a higher percentage of apoptosis in the seminal plasma of infertile men compared to healthy volunteers [8]. After adding 100 µmole of H_2O_2 to 12 semen samples to induce OS, Mahfouz et al. reported a higher percentage of apoptosis after H_2O_2 exposure [39]. Wang et al. compared semen samples from 35 patients with idiopathic infertility with 8 samples from healthy volunteers. The authors detected significantly higher levels of ROS (4.15×10^6 counted photons per minute [cpm] vs. 0.06×10^6 cpm; P .01), cytochrome C (2.78 vs. 1.5; P .01), caspase 9 (2.52 vs. 6; P .006), and caspase 3 (0.56 vs. 1.69; P .01) in infertile men vs. healthy volunteers, respectively [40].

1.4.2   ROS and Lipid Peroxidation

Lipid peroxidation (LPO) is the most extensively studied manifestation of ROS in biology. LPO is generally defined as oxidative induced damage of fatty acids that contain more than two carbon double bonds, also known as PUFA [41]. This is because most PUFA contain a double bond next to a methylene group weakening the methylene-carbon-hydrogen bond. As a result, free radicals are capable of capturing the hydrogen moiety from PUFA leaving an unpaired electron on the fatty acid that can be oxidized to form a peroxyl radical (Fig. 1.2). Lipid peroxides are unstable and decompose to form a complex series of compounds, which ultimately end up with MDA.

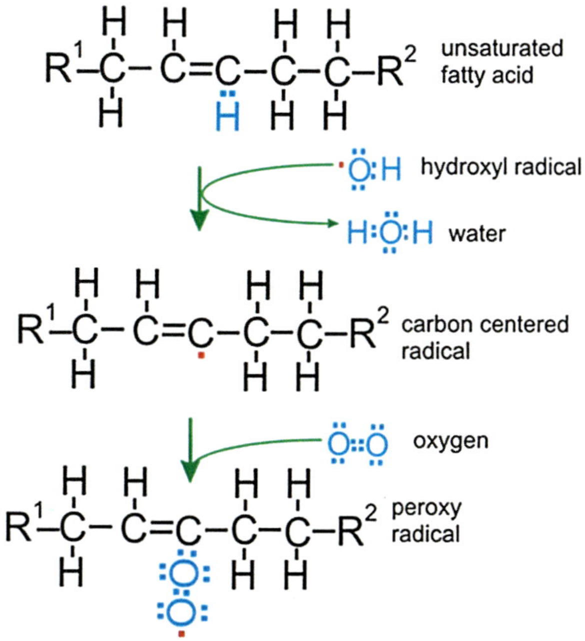

Fig. 1.2 Lipid peroxidation of polyunsaturated fatty acids (Self-created; no copyright)

LPO measurement relies on the interaction of MDA with thiobarbituric acid (TBA). While this method is controversial in that it is quite sensitive, but not necessarily specific to MDA, it remains the most widely used means to determine LPO. The resulting membrane structure disturbance affects vital functions such as signal transduction and maintenance of ion and metabolite gradient necessary for optimal sperm function. Unlike other cells, spermatozoa are unable to overcome the resulting damage since they lack the necessary cytoplasmic enzymes involved in the repair process [42].

1.4.3 ROS and Sperm Motility

Normal sperm motility is an integral requirement for male fertility. The free radical's ability to reduce sperm motility was first described by Jones et al. in 1979 [43], who linked ROS-induced LPO to reduction of sperm tail motion. ROS illicit a cascade of events that result in a decrease in axonemal protein phosphorylation and sperm immobilization [44]. H_2O_2 can inhibit the activity of G6PD decreasing the availability of NADPH thereby causing an accumulation of oxidized glutathione. The latter can reduce the antioxidant defenses of the spermatozoa which ultimately aggravate peroxidation of membrane phospholipids [44]. A direct cytotoxic effect for ROS on sperm mitochondria was also recognized as another cause for impaired sperm motility [27, 45, 46].

Clinical studies evaluating the link between ROS levels and defects in sperm motility have confirmed the presence of a negative association. du Plessis et al. [47] examined the influence of exogenous H_2O_2 addition to semen samples on sperm motility parameters and intracellular ROS and nitric oxide (NO) levels. After incubating human spermatozoa from ten donors with different exogenous H_2O_2 concentrations (0, 2.5, 7.5, and 15 µmole), they detected a significant inversely proportional relationship with sperm total motility (7.5 µmole 28.3 ± 4.01, $P < 0.001$; 15 µmole 16.67 ± 3.33, $P < 0.001$, versus control, 60.33 ± 6.86) and progressive motility (2.5 µmole 14 ± 1.65, $P < 0.01$; 7.5 µmole 10 ± 2.28, $P < 0.001$; 15 µmole 6.33 ± 1.68, $P < 0.001$, versus control, 29.33 ± 4.56). Higher concentrations of H_2O_2 significantly increased both NO (172.40 ± 22.341 % versus control; $P < 0.05$) and ROS levels (130.40 ± 7.108 % versus control; $P < 0.05$). The percentage of total motility was also inversely correlated with both endogenous NO ($r^2 = 0.99$, $P = 0.0041$) and ROS ($r^2 = 0.965$, $P = 0.017$) levels [47].

Urata et al. [48] incubated sperm from 37 healthy volunteers with lipopolysaccharide (LPS), an OS inducer, with and without antioxidant scavengers. Sperm motility was inhibited by 15 % in the presence of 0.1 µg/mL, 21 % in the presence of 1 µg/mL, and 50 % in the presence of 10 µg/mL dose of LPS after 60 minutes of incubation, compared with the control groups ($P < 0.05$). LPS-treated groups had a significantly higher ROS production in comparison to the control groups ($P < 0.05$). The addition of ROS scavengers such as superoxide dismutase and glutathione restored the motility index and suppressed ROS production in the LPS-treated semen samples [48]. Kourouma et al. [49] examined the in vitro administration of nonylphenol, a chemical known to induce OS by generating H_2O_2 and $\cdot O_2^-$, on epididymal sperm from 24 Sprague Dawley rats. Results showed a significant decline in the percentage of motile spermatozoa ($P < 0.001$) in a dose-related manner [49].

1.4.4 ROS and Sperm DNA Damage

Sperm DNA is uniquely structured to keep its nuclear chromatin highly stable, compact, and protected against assaults. It undergoes timely de-condensation to ensure the proper transfer of the packaged genetic material to the ovum during the fertilization process. Sperm DNA damage can occur as a consequence of OS and is thought to occur secondary to dysregulated apoptosis factors (Fig. 1.3). ROS can alter DNA integrity through modification of nucleic bases resulting in deletions, cross-links, frameshifts, and chromosomal rearrangements [50–52]. Such changes destabilize the DNA backbone, causing single- and double-strand DNA breaks [53]. The significance of sperm DNA fragmentation (SDF) has been acknowledged in male infertility. High SDF has been found to decrease the chances of natural pregnancy [54], increase the likelihood of miscarriages [55], and decrease the outcomes of assisted reproductive techniques, specifically intrauterine insemination [56] and conventional in vitro fertilization [57].

The relationship between OS and DNA damage has been proven in numerous reports. Lommiello et al. investigated semen samples from 56 infertile men and

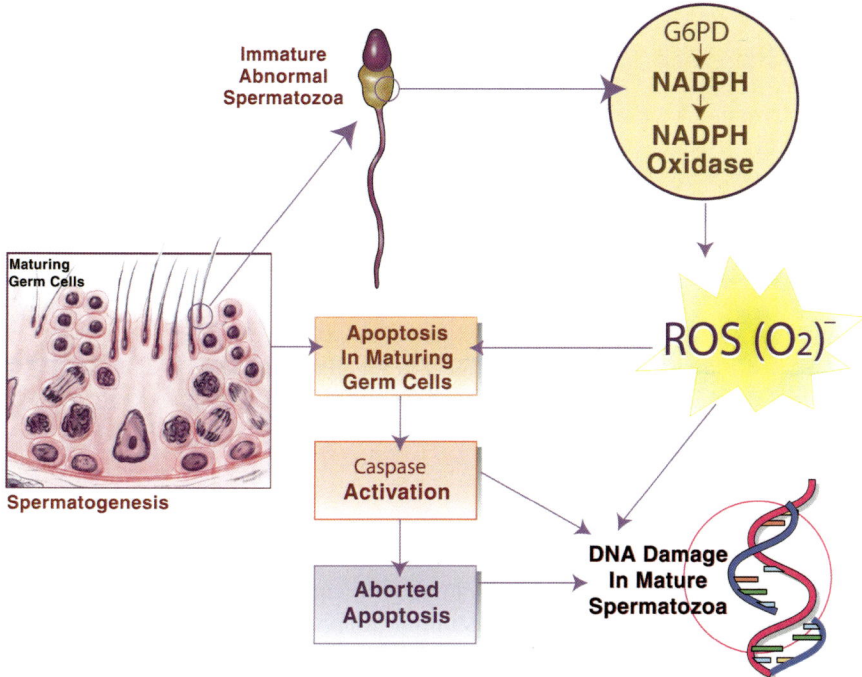

Fig. 1.3 OS-induced sperm DNA damage (Copyright license provided)

revealed a significant positive correlation between ROS levels and the degree of SDF ($p = 0.037$) [58]. In another study, semen collected from 63 patients attending an IVF unit was tested for physical characteristics along with ROS levels and SDF. The authors reported a strong positive correlation between intrinsic ROS levels and SDF measurements [59].

1.4.5   ROS in Varicocele

Varicocele is a common medical condition that has long been implicated as a major cause of male infertility [60, 61]. It is prevalent in about 15 % of the general male population, 35 % of men with primary infertility, and up to 80 % in men with secondary infertility [62, 63]. OS is now widely believed to be the common underlying pathophysiology causing infertility in varicocele patients [64, 65]. Studies involving OS markers in the semen of men with varicocele detected a significant increase of such markers in varicocele patients compared to controls [66].

Seminal ROS levels measured by chemiluminescence were significantly higher in infertile men with varicocele than fertile controls. Moreover, Allamaneni et al. [67] reported a positive correlation between seminal ROS levels and varicocele grade meaning that men with larger varicoceles had significantly higher seminal ROS levels than men with small varicoceles. Among healthy fertile men, the presence of varicocele was associated with a significant increase in ROS levels in comparison to men without varicocele [68]. Higher seminal levels of specific free radicals, namely, NO and NO synthase, have been detected in infertile men with varicocele compared with fertile men without varicocele [69–72]. Seminal levels of H_2O_2 and extracellular seminal O_2 were also found to be significantly higher in infertile men with varicocele in comparison to fertile healthy controls [73, 74].

Interestingly, surgical treatment of varicocele has been shown to reduce seminal OS in varicocele patients [75]. In one study, Sakamoto et al. [69] found that a time lag of approximately 6 months is required to achieve a marked improvement in seminal ROS markers after varicocele repair. Mostafa et al. [76] demonstrated a significant reduction of markers of seminal OS and an elevation of antioxidant levels 3 and 6 months after varicocele ligation. Finally, Hurtado de Catalfo et al. [77] reported normalization of seminal levels of antioxidant enzymes compared with age-matched fertile controls after varicocele ligation.

1.5 Measurement of ROS

Screening for OS is increasingly gaining attention in the evaluation of infertile men as current evidence has confirmed its utility in various clinical presentations [78]. ROS can be tested through direct or indirect assays (Table 1.1). Direct assays measure the amount of oxidation within the sperm cell membrane [79], while indirect assays estimate the detrimental effects of oxidative stress, such as DNA damage or lipid peroxidation levels [79]. The most commonly utilized methods for detection of ROS levels include:

1.5.1 Chemiluminescence Assay

This assay measures the oxidative end products of the interaction between ROS and certain reagents, which results in an emission of light that can be measured with a luminometer (Fig. 1.4) [80]. Two reagents are available, luminol and lucigenin. In contrast to lucigenin, which detects only the superoxide anion [81, 82], luminol has few advantages such as: (1) it has the ability to react with different ROS, including superoxide anion, hydroxyl radical, and hydrogen peroxide; (2) it measures both intra- and extracellular free radicals; and (3) it conducts a fast reaction allowing rapid measurement [83]. To ensure accurate readings, semen samples should contain sperm

Table 1.1 Types of ROS measurement assays

Direct assays	Indirect assays
Chemiluminescence	Total antioxidant capacity
Flow cytometry	Sperm DNA fragmentation
Nitroblue tetrazolium test	Chemokines
Thiobarbituric acid assay	Oxidation-reduction potential
Cytochrome C reduction test	Myeloperoxidase/Endtz test
Electron spin resonance	

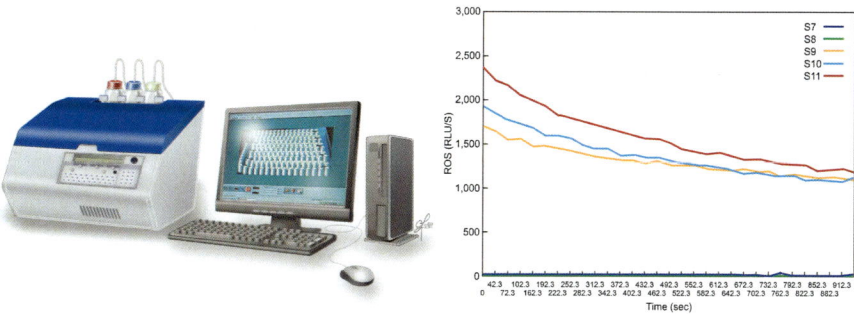

Fig. 1.4 ROS measurement by chemiluminescence assay: AutoLumat 953 Plus Luminometer connected to a computer with a sample result graph (Copyright license provided)

concentration $1 \times 10^6/mL$ or greater and be analyzed within the first hour of collection. Despite its clinical applicability, the widespread use of the chemiluminescence assay has been hampered by equipment expenses and the presence of assay confounders such as incubation time, leukocyte, and seminal plasma contamination [84].

1.5.2 Flow Cytometry

Flow cytometry is an alternative method that can also be used to measure intracellular sperm ROS [85]. It quantifies the amount of fluorescence per cell. Excited by a light source, cells emit light that is passed through optical filters before reaching optical detectors. Optical filters allow light of specific wavelengths to pass, thereby producing waves of specific colors. Flow cytometry is also an expensive tool that is not practical for widespread clinical use.

1.5.3 Nitroblue Tetrazolium (NBT) Assay

NBT is a cost-effective user-friendly assay. Using a light microscope, it can accurately predict ROS levels and provide insight on the potential source of OS, i.e., spermatozoa or leukocytes. It is based on the ability of NBT to interact with the superoxide present within spermatozoa or leukocytes converting into a blue pigment called diformazan, which can be measured and correlated with intracellular ROS concentration [78, 86].

1.5.4 Measurement of MDA Levels

The most commonly used method of assessing sperm membrane peroxidation is MDA level measurement via the TBA assay. Sensitive high-pressure liquid chromatography (HPLC) equipment [87, 88] or spectrofluorometric measurement of iron-based promoters [89] may be utilized for detection of the low sperm MDA concentrations. On the other hand, seminal plasma MDA levels are five to tenfold higher than sperm, making measurement with standard spectrophotometers possible [90]. The clinical relevance of MDA measurement emerges from its significant positive correlation with seminal ROS levels in men with infertility, compared with fertile controls or normozoospermic individuals [90–92]. Furthermore, in vitro studies have linked ROS-induced abnormalities in motility, sperm DNA integrity, and sperm-oocyte fusion with an increase in MDA concentration [33, 89].

1.5.5 Measurement of Oxidation-Reduction Potential

Oxidation-reduction potential (ORP), also known as the redox potential, is a measure of the potential for electrons to move from one chemical species to another [93]. ORP is a measure of this relationship between oxidants and antioxidants, providing a comprehensive measure of OS. Recently, a novel technology based on a galvanostatic measure of electrons has been developed (MiOXSYS) and utilized to evaluate changes in OS in trauma patients and as a function of extreme exercise [94–96]. The MiOXSYS is a simple, rapid, and inexpensive system composed of the analyzer and disposable test sensor (Fig. 1.5). It measures the electron transfer from reductants (antioxidants) to oxidants under a steady low-voltage reducing current. Thus, it provides an aggregate measure of all current oxidant activity and antioxidant activity in a sample. Higher ORP values (millivolts, mV) indicate a higher

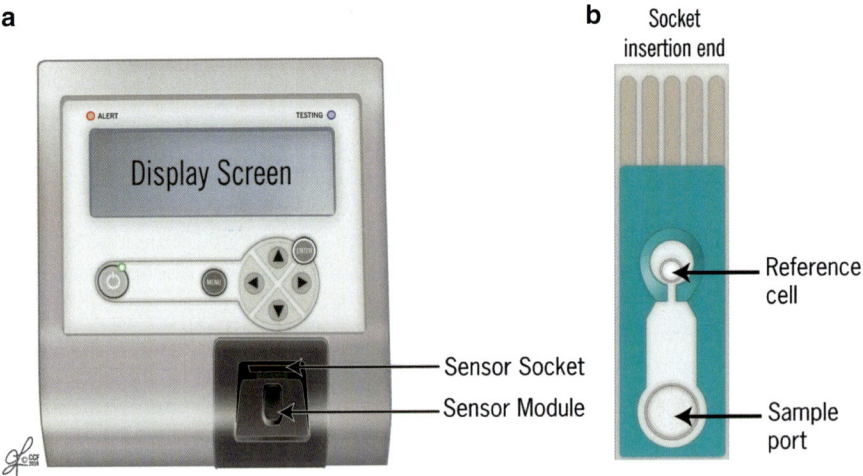

Fig. 1.5 The MiOXSYS System comprises an (**a**) analyzer and (**b**) a disposable sensor (Copyright license provided)

oxidant activity relative to the antioxidant activity and therefore greater state of OS. Recent studies have confirmed the reliability of the MiOXSYS System in measuring ORP levels in semen and seminal plasma demonstrating the presence of significant negative correlations between ORP results and abnormalities of semen parameters [97].

1.5.6 Predictors of OS in Semen Studies

A number of routine laboratory tests have been suggested as possible predictors for the presence of OS in the semen [98]. While any abnormality in routine semen parameters (count, motility, morphology) may be associated with OS, asthenozoospermia is probably the best surrogate marker for OS in a routine semen analysis [99, 100]. The presence of an exaggerated number of round cells in the semen may represent leukocytes and hence possible OS [26]. These cells, however, may represent immature germ cells and hence need to be tested with ancillary tests such as peroxidase test, CD45 staining, or measurement of seminal elastase activity [101, 102]. Poor sperm viability detected by the hypoosmotic swelling test or dye exclusion assays has been linked with the presence of sperm OS [103]. Additionally, macroscopic semen parameters have also been considered. Hyperviscosity of the seminal plasma, an observation that is commonly seen with infection, has been linked to increased levels of seminal plasma MDA [104] and reduced seminal plasma antioxidant status [105].

1.6 Management of OS

OS management is based on alleviating potential causes of excessive ROS production or boosting the patient's antioxidant system to counterbalance the hazardous effects of ROS.

1.6.1 Lifestyle Modification

The accompanying stresses of the modern world have caused an increase in negative behaviors such as smoking, substance abuse, and obesity, all of which have been shown to contribute to OS, and, therefore, minimizing such unfavorable behavior is likely to aid in alleviating OS [106].

Environmental exposures to heat, pollution, toxins, and heavy metals should be minimized as these can result in development of OS. Moreover, activities capable of increasing scrotal temperature such as hot baths, saunas, extended periods of driving, and long and sedentary office hours should be avoided. Finally, adequate protective equipment and aeration should be ensured at workplaces to limit exposure to any chemical or vapor that may cause OS.

1.6.2 Treatment of Potential Sources of ROS

As stated previously, leukocytospermia is a significant source of ROS in seminal plasma. A significant association between leukocytospermia and genitourinary infection has been acknowledged [107], which, if confirmed by a positive culture, should be treated with appropriate antibiotics. Controversy regarding the value of treating asymptomatic leukocytospermia in infertile men exists and stems from the fact that spontaneous improvement of seminal WBC levels has been witnessed in about 40 % of cases [108]. Anti-inflammatory medications (Cox-2 inhibitors) and broad-spectrum antibiotics (doxycycline, erythromycin, and trimethoprim/sulfamethoxazole) have been tried successfully reducing seminal WBC levels and improving semen parameters [109, 110].

Varicocele is another condition eliciting OS [66, 75]. In addition to the favorable influence varicocele ligation has on semen parameters [111], a decrease in seminal ROS levels has invariably been demonstrated, thereby protecting the sperm membrane and DNA from oxidative damage [66, 98].

1.6.3 Antioxidant Supplementation

Antioxidants work by stopping the oxidation cascade through scavenging, neutralizing, or reducing the formation of ROS [45]. There are two types of antioxidants: (1) preventive antioxidants, which are chelators or binding proteins that prevent the formation of ROS, and (2) scavenging antioxidants, such as vitamins C and E, which can quench the ROS that is already present [112].

A number of systematic reviews have explored available evidence on antioxidant use yielding variable conclusions. A Cochrane review of 48 randomized controlled clinical trials including 4179 subfertile men was recently performed [113]. Live birth and pregnancy rates were reported in four and seven trials, respectively. Despite a considerable variability in the reported antioxidant effect on semen parameters, a statistically significant improvement in live birth rate (OR 4.21, 95 % CI 2.08 to 8.51; $P < 0.0001$) and clinical pregnancy rate (OR 3.43, 95 % CI 1.92 to 6.11; $P < 0.0001$) was detected [113].

Different selection criteria were utilized in other literature reviews. Ross et al. [114] analyzed 17 randomized trials, including a total of 1665 infertile men on whom oral antioxidants were compared to placebo or no treatment. Semen parameters and reported pregnancy rates were the outcome measures analyzed. Despite the methodological and clinical heterogeneity, an improvement in sperm after antioxidant therapy was reported in 14 out of 17 trials. Pregnancy rate was reported in seven trials, six of them showed a significant improvement after antioxidant therapy. The authors concluded that the use of oral antioxidants in infertile men may have a beneficial effect on sperm quality and pregnancy rates.

In an attempt to evaluate the impact of oral antioxidants on measures of sperm oxidative stress and DNA damage, Gharagozloo and Aitken selected 20 trials that assessed such an association [115]. Analysis showed that 19 out of the 20 studies reported a significant reduction of oxidative stress or DNA damage after treatments with antioxidants. Moreover, an improvement in sperm motility, particularly in asthenozoospermic patients, was significantly observed [115]. In addition to addressing the effect of oral antioxidants on sperm dysfunction and DNA damage, Zini and Al-Hathal also investigated the in vitro use of antioxidants prior to assisted reproduction revealing a protective effect for antioxidants against exogenous ROS, sperm cryopreservation, and thawing [112].

Although many reviews generally demonstrate a favorable influence for antioxidants on male fertility, the ideal regimen of antioxidants is still unknown. This is mainly due to the lack of knowledge of what is a normal redox level in the human body. Currently, no generally accepted normal values for this important parameter exist. In addition, many patients are taking antioxidants in an uncontrolled manner, which in turn might shift the fine balance that is essential for normal sperm function from the OS or normal levels into the so-called reductive stress, which is as dangerous as OS and can be the cause of cancer and heart or neurological disease including infertility among others [116–119]. Many experts suggest an individualized treatment approach where the dose and type of antioxidant should be adjusted according to the clinical presentation and/or the level of seminal oxidative stress.

Conclusion

ROS play a vital role in male reproduction. At low levels, they ensure optimal sperm function necessary for fertilization and embryo development. However, when excessive amounts of ROS are produced, they can inflict undesirable effects such as aggravated apoptosis, lipid peroxidation, and DNA damage ultimately worsening sperm function and causing infertility. Measuring seminal ROS levels should become an integral part of male fertility evaluation as it can guide clinicians with their management strategies and provide a sound modality for patient follow-up.

References

1. Cooper TG et al. World Health Organization reference values for human semen characteristics. Hum Reprod Update. 2010;16:231–45. doi:10.1093/humupd/dmp048.
2. Poongothai J, Gopenath TS, Manonayaki S. Genetics of human male infertility. Singapore Med J. 2009;50:336–47.
3. Agarwal A et al. Reactive oxygen species as an independent marker of male factor infertility. Fertil Steril. 2006;86:878–85. doi:10.1016/j.fertnstert.2006.02.111.
4. Agarwal A, Virk G, Ong C, du Plessis SS. Effect of oxidative stress on male reproduction. World J Mens Health. 2014;32:1–17. doi:10.5534/wjmh.2014.32.1.1.
5. Lanzafame FM, La Vignera S, Vicari E, Calogero AE. Oxidative stress and medical antioxidant treatment in male infertility. Reprod Biomed Online. 2009;19:638–59.
6. Padron OF et al. Seminal reactive oxygen species and sperm motility and morphology in men with spinal cord injury. Fertil Steril. 1997;67:1115–20.
7. Aziz N, Agarwal A, Lewis-Jones I, Sharma RK, Thomas Jr AJ. Novel associations between specific sperm morphological defects and leukocytospermia. Fertil Steril. 2004;82:621–7. doi:10.1016/j.fertnstert.2004.02.112.

8. Moustafa MH et al. Relationship between ROS production, apoptosis and DNA denaturation in spermatozoa from patients examined for infertility. Hum Reprod. 2004;19:129–38.
9. Alvarez JG, Storey BT. Differential incorporation of fatty acids into and peroxidative loss of fatty acids from phospholipids of human spermatozoa. Mol Reprod Dev. 1995;42:334–46. doi:10.1002/mrd.1080420311.
10. Aitken RJ, Roman SD. Antioxidant systems and oxidative stress in the testes. Adv Exp Med Biol. 2008;636:154–71. doi:10.1007/978-0-387-09597-4_9.
11. Halliwell B. Free radicals and vascular disease: how much do we know? BMJ. 1993;307: 885–6.
12. Lobascio AM et al. Involvement of seminal leukocytes, reactive oxygen species, and sperm mitochondrial membrane potential in the DNA damage of the human spermatozoa. Andrology. 2015;3:265–70. doi:10.1111/andr.302.
13. Koppers AJ, De Iuliis GN, Finnie JM, McLaughlin EA, Aitken RJ. Significance of mitochondrial reactive oxygen species in the generation of oxidative stress in spermatozoa. J Clin Endocrinol Metab. 2008;93:3199–207. doi:10.1210/jc.2007-2616.
14. Gil-Guzman E et al. Differential production of reactive oxygen species by subsets of human spermatozoa at different stages of maturation. Hum Reprod. 2001;16:1922–30.
15. Tanphaichitr N et al. Remodeling of the plasma membrane in preparation for sperm-egg recognition: roles of acrosomal proteins. Asian J Androl. 2015;17:574–82. doi:10.4103/1008-682X.152817.
16. Aitken RJ, Baker MA. Reactive oxygen species generation by human spermatozoa: a continuing enigma. Int J Androl. 2002;25:191–4.
17. Alani GT, El Yaseen HD. Creatine kinase activity and malondialdehyde in the seminal plasma of normospermic infertile males. Fac Med Baghdad. 2009;51:336–40.
18. Hallak J et al. Creatine kinase as an indicator of sperm quality and maturity in men with oligospermia. Urology. 2001;58:446–51.
19. Schatten H, Sun QY, Prather R. The impact of mitochondrial function/dysfunction on IVF and new treatment possibilities for infertility. Reprod Biol Endocrinol. 2014;12:111. doi:10.1186/1477-7827-12-111.
20. Griveau JF, Le Lannou D. Reactive oxygen species and human spermatozoa: physiology and pathology. Int J Androl. 1997;20:61–9.
21. Ayala A, Munoz MF, Arguelles S. Lipid peroxidation: production, metabolism, and signaling mechanisms of malondialdehyde and 4-hydroxy-2-nonenal. Oxid Med Cell Longev. 2014;2014:360438. doi:10.1155/2014/360438.
22. Sandoval JS, Raburn D, Mausher S. Leukocytospermia: overview of diagnosis, implications, and management of a controversial finding. Middle East Fertil Soc J. 2013;18:129–34.
23. World Health O. Laboratory manual of the WHO for the examination of human semen and sperm-cervical mucus interaction. Ann Ist Super Sanita. 2001;37:I–XII, 1–123.
24. Mupfiga C, Fisher D, Kruger T, Henkel R. The relationship between seminal leukocytes, oxidative status in the ejaculate, and apoptotic markers in human spermatozoa. Syst Biol Reprod Med. 2013;59:304–11. doi:10.3109/19396368.2013.821540.
25. Saleh RA et al. Leukocytospermia is associated with increased reactive oxygen species production by human spermatozoa. Fertil Steril. 2002;78:1215–24.
26. Sharma RK, Pasqualotto AE, Nelson DR, Thomas Jr AJ, Agarwal A. Relationship between seminal white blood cell counts and oxidative stress in men treated at an infertility clinic. J Androl. 2001;22:575–83.
27. de Lamirande E, Jiang H, Zini A, Kodama H, Gagnon C. Reactive oxygen species and sperm physiology. Rev Reprod. 1997;2:48–54.
28. Aitken RJ, Paterson M, Fisher H, Buckingham DW, van Duin M. Redox regulation of tyrosine phosphorylation in human spermatozoa and its role in the control of human sperm function. J Cell Sci. 1995;108(Pt 5):2017–25.
29. de Lamirande E, Gagnon C. Impact of reactive oxygen species on spermatozoa: a balancing act between beneficial and detrimental effects. Hum Reprod. 1995;10(Suppl 1):15–21.

30. Zini A, De Lamirande E, Gagnon C. Low levels of nitric oxide promote human sperm capacitation in vitro. J Androl. 1995;16:424–31.
31. Rivlin J, Mendel J, Rubinstein S, Etkovitz N, Breitbart H. Role of hydrogen peroxide in sperm capacitation and acrosome reaction. Biol Reprod. 2004;70:518–22. doi:10.1095/biolreprod.103.020487.
32. Aitken RJ, Harkiss D, Knox W, Paterson M, Irvine DS. A novel signal transduction cascade in capacitating human spermatozoa characterised by a redox-regulated, cAMP-mediated induction of tyrosine phosphorylation. J Cell Sci. 1998;111(Pt 5):645–56.
33. Aitken RJ, Clarkson JS, Fishel S. Generation of reactive oxygen species, lipid peroxidation, and human sperm function. Biol Reprod. 1989;41:183–97.
34. Print CG, Loveland KL. Germ cell suicide: new insights into apoptosis during spermatogenesis. Bioessays. 2000;22:423–30. doi:10.1002/(SICI)1521-1878(200005)22:5<423::AID-BIES4>3.0.CO;2-0.
35. Hikim AP et al. Spontaneous germ cell apoptosis in humans: evidence for ethnic differences in the susceptibility of germ cells to programmed cell death. J Clin Endocrinol Metab. 1998;83:152–6. doi:10.1210/jcem.83.1.4485.
36. Fathi Najafi T et al. Assessment of sperm apoptosis and semen quality in infertile men-meta analysis. Iran Red Crescent Med J. 2012;14:182–3.
37. Sakkas D, Mariethoz E, St John JC. Abnormal sperm parameters in humans are indicative of an abortive apoptotic mechanism linked to the Fas-mediated pathway. Exp Cell Res. 1999;251:350–5. doi:10.1006/excr.1999.4586.
38. Henkel, R. DNA fragmentation and its influence on fertilization and pregnancy outcome. in: S.C. Oehninger, T.F. Kruger (Eds.) Male infertility: diagnosis and treatment. Informa Healthcare, London, UK; 2007:277–90.
39. Mahfouz RZ et al. Sperm viability, apoptosis, and intracellular reactive oxygen species levels in human spermatozoa before and after induction of oxidative stress. Fertil Steril. 2010;93:814–21. doi:10.1016/j.fertnstert.2008.10.068.
40. Wang X et al. Oxidative stress is associated with increased apoptosis leading to spermatozoa DNA damage in patients with male factor infertility. Fertil Steril. 2003;80:531–5.
41. Halliwell B. How to characterize a biological antioxidant. Free Radic Res Commun. 1990;9:1–32.
42. Agarwal A, Saleh RA, Bedaiwy MA. Role of reactive oxygen species in the pathophysiology of human reproduction. Fertil Steril. 2003;79:829–43.
43. Jones R, Mann T, Sherins R. Peroxidative breakdown of phospholipids in human spermatozoa, spermicidal properties of fatty acid peroxides and protective action of seminal plasma. Fertil Steril. 1979;31:531–7.
44. Aitken RJ. Molecular mechanisms regulating human sperm function. Mol Hum Reprod. 1997;3:169–73.
45. Bansal AK, Bilaspuri GS. Impacts of oxidative stress and antioxidants on semen functions. Vet Med Int. 2010; doi:10.4061/2011/686137.
46. Aitken RJ, Jones KT, Robertson SA. Reactive oxygen species and sperm function--in sickness and in health. J Androl. 2012;33:1096–106. doi:10.2164/jandrol.112.016535.
47. du Plessis SS et al. Effects of H(2)O(2) exposure on human sperm motility parameters, reactive oxygen species levels and nitric oxide levels. Andrologia. 2010;42:206–10. doi:10.1111/j.1439-0272.2009.00980.x.
48. Urata K et al. Effect of endotoxin-induced reactive oxygen species on sperm motility. Fertil Steril. 2001;76:163–6.
49. Kourouma A. et al. In vitro assessment of ROS on motility of epididymal sperm of male rat exposed to intraperitoneal administration of nonylphenol Asian Pacific Journal of Reproduction. 2015;4:169–78.
50. Kemal Duru N, Morshedi M, Oehninger S. Effects of hydrogen peroxide on DNA and plasma membrane integrity of human spermatozoa. Fertil Steril. 2000;74:1200–7.
51. Sharma RK, Said T, Agarwal A. Sperm DNA damage and its clinical relevance in assessing reproductive outcome. Asian J Androl. 2004;6:139–48.

52. Thomson LK et al. Cryopreservation-induced human sperm DNA damage is predominantly mediated by oxidative stress rather than apoptosis. Hum Reprod. 2009;24:2061–70. doi:10.1093/humrep/dep214.
53. Aitken RJ, Krausz C. Oxidative stress. DNA damage and the Y chromosome. Reproduction. 2001;122:497–506.
54. Evenson DP et al. Utility of the sperm chromatin structure assay as a diagnostic and prognostic tool in the human fertility clinic. Hum Reprod. 1999;14:1039–49.
55. Khadem N, Poorhoseyni A, Jalali M, Akbary A, Heydari ST. Sperm DNA fragmentation in couples with unexplained recurrent spontaneous abortions. Andrologia. 2014;46:126–30. doi:10.1111/and.12056.
56. Duran EH, Morshedi M, Taylor S, Oehninger S. Sperm DNA quality predicts intrauterine insemination outcome: a prospective cohort study. Hum Reprod. 2002;17:3122–8.
57. Zini A, Sigman M. Are tests of sperm DNA damage clinically useful? Pros and cons. J Androl. 2009;30:219–29. doi:10.2164/jandrol.108.006908.
58. Iommiello VM et al. Ejaculate oxidative stress is related with sperm DNA fragmentation and round cells. Int J Endocrinol. 2015;321901:2015. doi:10.1155/2015/321901.
59. Henkel R et al. Effect of reactive oxygen species produced by spermatozoa and leukocytes on sperm functions in non-leukocytospermic patients. Fertil Steril. 2005;83:635–42. doi:10.1016/j.fertnstert.2004.11.022.
60. Majzoub A, Esteves SC, Gosalvez J, Agarwal A. Specialized sperm function tests in varicocele and the future of andrology laboratory. Asian J Androl. 2016;18:205–12. doi:10.4103/1008-682X.172642.
61. Agarwal A, Esteves SC. Varicocele and male infertility: current concepts and future perspectives. Asian J Androl. 2016;18:161–2. doi:10.4103/1008-682X.172819.
62. Pfeiffer D, Berger J, Schoop C, Tauber R. A Doppler-based study on the prevalence of varicocele in German children and adolescents. Andrologia. 2006;38:13–9. doi:10.1111/j.1439-0272.2006.00680.x.
63. ElBardisi H, et al. Varicocele among infertile men in Qatar. Andrologia. 2016. doi:10.1111/and.12637.
64. Mancini A et al. Biochemical alterations in semen of varicocele patients: a review of the literature. Adv Urol. 2012;2012:903931. doi:10.1155/2012/903931.
65. Cho CL, Esteves SC, Agarwal A. Novel insights into the pathophysiology of varicocele and its association with reactive oxygen species and sperm DNA fragmentation. Asian J Androl. 2016;18:186–93. doi:10.4103/1008-682X.170441.
66. Agarwal A, Hamada A, Esteves SC. Insight into oxidative stress in varicocele-associated male infertility: part 1. Nature reviews. Urology. 2012;9:678–90. doi:10.1038/nrurol.2012.197.
67. Allamaneni SS, Naughton CK, Sharma RK, Thomas Jr AJ, Agarwal A. Increased seminal reactive oxygen species levels in patients with varicoceles correlate with varicocele grade but not with testis size. Fertil Steril. 2004;82:1684–6. doi:10.1016/j.fertnstert.2004.04.071.
68. Mostafa T, Anis T, Imam H, El-Nashar AR, Osman IA. Seminal reactive oxygen species-antioxidant relationship in fertile males with and without varicocele. Andrologia. 2009;41:125–9. doi:10.1111/j.1439-0272.2008.00900.x.
69. Sakamoto Y, Ishikawa T, Kondo Y, Yamaguchi K, Fujisawa M. The assessment of oxidative stress in infertile patients with varicocele. BJU international. 2008;101:1547–52. doi:10.1111/j.1464-410X.2008.07517.x.
70. Mehraban D et al. Comparison of nitric oxide concentration in seminal fluid between infertile patients with and without varicocele and normal fertile men. Urology journal. 2005;2:106–10.
71. Xu Y, Xu QY, Yang BH, Zhu XM, Peng YF. Relationship of nitric oxide and nitric oxide synthase with varicocele infertility. Zhonghua nan ke xue. 2008;14:414–7.
72. Abd-Elmoaty MA, Saleh R, Sharma R, Agarwal A. Increased levels of oxidants and reduced antioxidants in semen of infertile men with varicocele. Fertil Steril. 2010;94:1531–4. doi:10.1016/j.fertnstert.2009.12.039.

73. Mostafa T, Anis T, El Nashar A, Imam H, Osman I. Seminal plasma reactive oxygen species-antioxidants relationship with varicocele grade. Andrologia. 2012;44:66–9. doi:10.1111/j.1439-0272.2010.01111.x.
74. Mazzilli F, Rossi T, Marchesini M, Ronconi C, Dondero F. Superoxide anion in human semen related to seminal parameters and clinical aspects. Fertil Steril. 1994;62:862–8.
75. Hamada A, Esteves SC, Agarwal A. Insight into oxidative stress in varicocele-associated male infertility: part 2. Nature reviews. Urology. 2013;10:26–37. doi:10.1038/nrurol.2012.198.
76. Mostafa T, Anis TH, El-Nashar A, Imam H, Othman IA. Varicocelectomy reduces reactive oxygen species levels and increases antioxidant activity of seminal plasma from infertile men with varicocele. Int J Androl. 2001;24:261–5.
77. Hurtado de Catalfo GE, Ranieri-Casilla A, Marra FA, de Alaniz MJ, Marra CA. Oxidative stress biomarkers and hormonal profile in human patients undergoing varicocelectomy. Int J Androl. 2007;30:519–30. doi:10.1111/j.1365-2605.2007.00753.x.
78. Agarwal A, Makker K, Sharma R. Clinical relevance of oxidative stress in male factor infertility: an update. Am J Reprod Immunol. 2008;59:2–11. doi:10.1111/j.1600-0897.2007.00559.x.
79. Agarwal A, Tvrda E, Sharma R. Relationship amongst teratozoospermia, seminal oxidative stress and male infertility. Reprod Biol Endocrinol. 2014;12:45. doi:10.1186/1477-7827-12-45.
80. Athayde KS et al. Development of normal reference values for seminal reactive oxygen species and their correlation with leukocytes and semen parameters in a fertile population. J Androl. 2007;28:613–20. doi:10.2164/jandrol.106.001966.
81. Li Y, Stansbury KH, Zhu H, Trush MA. Biochemical characterization of lucigenin (Bis-N-methylacridinium) as a chemiluminescent probe for detecting intramitochondrial superoxide anion radical production. Biochem Biophys Res Commun. 1999;262:80–7. doi:10.1006/bbrc.1999.1174.
82. McKinney KA, Lewis SE, Thompson W. Reactive oxygen species generation in human sperm: luminol and lucigenin chemiluminescence probes. Arch Androl. 1996;36:119–25.
83. Aitken RJ, Buckingham DW, West KM. Reactive oxygen species and human spermatozoa: analysis of the cellular mechanisms involved in luminol- and lucigenin-dependent chemiluminescence. J Cell Physiol. 1992;151:466–77. doi:10.1002/jcp.1041510305.
84. Aitken RJ, Baker MA, O'Bryan M. Shedding light on chemiluminescence: the application of chemiluminescence in diagnostic andrology. J Androl. 2004;25:455–65.
85. Guthrie HD, Welch GR. Using fluorescence-activated flow cytometry to determine reactive oxygen species formation and membrane lipid peroxidation in viable boar spermatozoa. Methods Mol Biol. 2010;594:163–71. doi:10.1007/978-1-60761-411-1_12.
86. Kefer JC, Agarwal A, Sabanegh E. Role of antioxidants in the treatment of male infertility. Int J Urol. 2009;16:449–57. doi:10.1111/j.1442-2042.2009.02280.x.
87. Shang XJ et al. Analysis of lipid peroxidative levels in seminal plasma of infertile men by high-performance liquid chromatography. Arch Androl. 2004;50:411–6.
88. Li K, Shang X, Chen Y. High-performance liquid chromatographic detection of lipid peroxidation in human seminal plasma and its application to male infertility. Clin Chim Acta. 2004;346:199–203. doi:10.1016/j.cccn.2004.03.013.
89. Aitken RJ, Harkiss D, Buckingham D. Relationship between iron-catalysed lipid peroxidation potential and human sperm function. J Reprod Fertil. 1993;98:257–65.
90. Tavilani H, Doosti M, Saeidi H. Malondialdehyde levels in sperm and seminal plasma of asthenozoospermic and its relationship with semen parameters. Clin Chim Acta. 2005;356:199–203. doi:10.1016/j.cccn.2005.01.017.
91. Nakamura H et al. Detection of oxidative stress in seminal plasma and fractionated sperm from subfertile male patients. Eur J Obstet Gynecol Reprod Biol. 2002;105:155–60.
92. Hsieh YY, Chang CC, Lin CS. Seminal malondialdehyde concentration but not glutathione peroxidase activity is negatively correlated with seminal concentration and motility. Int J Biol Sci. 2006;2:23–9.
93. McCord JM. The evolution of free radicals and oxidative stress. Am J Med. 2000;108:652–9.

94. Rael LT et al. Plasma oxidation-reduction potential and protein oxidation in traumatic brain injury. J Neurotrauma. 2009;26:1203–11. doi:10.1089/neu.2008-0816.
95. Rael LT et al. Oxidation-reduction potential and paraoxonase-arylesterase activity in trauma patients. Biochem Biophys Res Commun. 2007;361:561–5. doi:10.1016/j.bbrc.2007.07.078.
96. Stagos D et al. Application of a new oxidation-reduction potential assessment method in strenuous exercise-induced oxidative stress. Redox Rep. 2015;20:154–62. doi:10.1179/1351000214Y.0000000118.
97. Agarwal A, Sharma R, Roychoudhury S, Du Plessis S, Sabanegh E. MiOXSYS: a novel method of measuring oxidation reduction potential in semen and seminal plasma. Fertil Steril. 2016; doi:10.1016/j.fertnstert.2016.05.013.
98. Tremellen K. Oxidative stress and male infertility--a clinical perspective. Hum Reprod Update. 2008;14:243–58. doi:10.1093/humupd/dmn004.
99. Keskes-Ammar L et al. Sperm oxidative stress and the effect of an oral vitamin E and selenium supplement on semen quality in infertile men. Arch Androl. 2003;49:83–94.
100. Kao SH et al. Increase of oxidative stress in human sperm with lower motility. Fertil Steril. 2008;89:1183–90. doi:10.1016/j.fertnstert.2007.05.029.
101. Zorn B, Sesek-Briski A, Osredkar J, Meden-Vrtovec H. Semen polymorphonuclear neutrophil leukocyte elastase as a diagnostic and prognostic marker of genital tract inflammation--a review. Clin Chem Lab Med. 2003;41:2–12. doi:10.1515/CCLM.2003.002.
102. Kopa Z, Wenzel J, Papp GK, Haidl G. Role of granulocyte elastase and interleukin-6 in the diagnosis of male genital tract inflammation. Andrologia. 2005;37:188–94. doi:10.1111/j.1439-0272.2005.00676.x.
103. Dandekar SP, Nadkarni GD, Kulkarni VS, Punekar S. Lipid peroxidation and antioxidant enzymes in male infertility. J Postgrad Med. 2002;48:186–9. ; discussion 189–90.
104. Aydemir B, Onaran I, Kiziler AR, Alici B, Akyolcu MC. The influence of oxidative damage on viscosity of seminal fluid in infertile men. J Androl. 2008;29:41–6. doi:10.2164/jandrol.107.003046.
105. Siciliano L et al. Impaired seminal antioxidant capacity in human semen with hyperviscosity or oligoasthenozoospermia. J Androl. 2001;22:798–803.
106. Wright C, Milne S, Leeson H. Sperm DNA damage caused by oxidative stress: modifiable clinical, lifestyle and nutritional factors in male infertility. Reprod Biomed Online. 2014;28:684–703. doi:10.1016/j.rbmo.2014.02.004.
107. Weidner W, Krause W, Ludwig M. Relevance of male accessory gland infection for subsequent fertility with special focus on prostatitis. Hum Reprod Update. 1999;5:421–32.
108. Lackner JE, Lakovic E, Waldhor T, Schatzl G, Marberger M. Spontaneous variation of leukocytospermia in asymptomatic infertile males. Fertil Steril. 2008;90:1757–60. doi:10.1016/j.fertnstert.2007.08.041.
109. Gambera L et al. Sperm quality and pregnancy rate after COX-2 inhibitor therapy of infertile males with abacterial leukocytospermia. Hum Reprod. 2007;22:1047–51. doi:10.1093/humrep/del490.
110. Skau PA, Folstad I. Do bacterial infections cause reduced ejaculatequality? A meta-analysis of antibiotic treatment of male infertility. Behav Ecol. 2003;14:40–7.
111. Majzoub A et al. Does the number of veins ligated during varicococele surgery influence post-operative semen and hormone results? Andrology. 2016; doi:10.1111/andr.12226.
112. Zini A, Al-Hathal N. Antioxidant therapy in male infertility: fact or fiction? Asian J Androl. 2011;13:374–81. doi:10.1038/aja.2010.182.
113. Showell MG, et al. Antioxidants for male subfertility. Cochrane Database Syst Rev. 2014;CD007411. doi:10.1002/14651858.CD007411.pub3.
114. Ross C et al. A systematic review of the effect of oral antioxidants on male infertility. Reprod Biomed Online. 2010;20:711–23. doi:10.1016/j.rbmo.2010.03.008.
115. Gharagozloo P, Aitken RJ. The role of sperm oxidative stress in male infertility and the significance of oral antioxidant therapy. Hum Reprod. 2011;26:1628–40. doi:10.1093/humrep/der132.

116. Henkel RR. Leukocytes and oxidative stress: dilemma for sperm function and male fertility. Asian J Androl. 2011;13:43–52. doi:10.1038/aja.2010.76.
117. Ufer C, Wang CC, Borchert A, Heydeck D, Kuhn H. Redox control in mammalian embryo development. Antioxid Redox Signal. 2010;13:833–75. doi:10.1089/ars.2009.3044.
118. Brewer AC, Mustafi SB, Murray TV, Rajasekaran NS, Benjamin IJ. Reductive stress linked to small HSPs, G6PD, and Nrf2 pathways in heart disease. Antioxid Redox Signal. 2013;18:1114–27. doi:10.1089/ars.2012.4914.
119. Lipinski B. Evidence in support of a concept of reductive stress. Br J Nutr. 2002;87:93–4; discussion 94. doi:10.1079/BJN2001435.

Biochemistry of Coenzyme Q10

2

Gian Paolo Littarru, Francesca Bruge, and Luca Tiano

2.1 Introduction

Coenzyme Q (CoQ) is a lipophilic quinone widely distributed in nature. The first homologue to be discovered about 50 years ago, in beef mitochondria, was coenzyme Q10 by Dr. P.L. Crane [8]. From those early studies, the essential coenzymatic activity in mitochondrial bioenergetics was soon recognized. CoQ is made of benzoquinone moiety and an isoprenoid side chain, the length of which is 10 units both in man and many mammals. Other living organisms possess different species of CoQ, for instance, *Saccharomyces cerevisiae* produces CoQ6, other microorganisms CoQ7 and many mammals CoQ9. Each organism possesses a dominant homologue of CoQ and minor amounts of other homologues; differently from other isoprenylated compounds introduced in the diet, such as menaquinones, the elongation of a certain CoQ homologue to CoQ10 is not possible. Most of the coenzyme Q10 in our organism is endogenously produced, although a small amount is ingested daily through the diet where it is present mainly in meat and fish and to a lower extent in some vegetables for an average intake of 5 mg/day. For this reason, being an endogenous cofactor

and hence not essential, but partially taken with the diet, it is also referred as a vitamin-like molecule.

Coenzyme Q10 is also known as ubiquinone because of its widespread, ubiquitous diffusion in living organisms [29]. This name was coniated by Dr. R.A. Morton, who also isolated and studied the compound in the early years of its discovery.

For a certain number of years, CoQ was mainly known for its key role in mitochondrial bioenergetics; later studies demonstrated its presence in other subcellular

G.P. Littarru • F. Bruge • L. Tiano (✉)
Department of Clinical and Dental Sciences – Biochemistry Section,
Polytechnic University of Marche, Ancona, Italy
e-mail: l.tiano@univpm.it

© Springer International Publishing Switzerland 2017
G. Balercia et al. (eds.), *Antioxidants in Andrology*, Trends in Andrology
and Sexual Medicine, DOI 10.1007/978-3-319-41749-3_2

fractions and in plasma and extensively investigated its antioxidant role. The rationale supporting the use of CoQ10 as a food supplement is mainly based on these two functions. At the inner mitochondrial membrane level, ubiquinone is also recognized as a cofactor for the function of uncoupling proteins and a modulator of the transition pore [9]. More recent data reveal that CoQ10 affects the expression of genes involved in human cell signalling, metabolism and transport [15], and some of the effects of exogenously administered CoQ10 may be due to this property. New progress has been made in elucidating CoQ10 in metabolism and nutrition. This short chapter focusses on basic biochemical mechanisms of CoQ10 in order to provide a background to better understand the relationship between those and phys-iological and clinical effects, with particular relevance to reproductive health.

2.2   CoQ10 and Mitochondrial Bioenergetics

The discovery of the CoQ10 molecule came about as a result of an intensive programme of research developed by Prof. D.E. Green, at the University of Wisconsin, to find out how mitochondria work. This occurred in 1957. It soon became evident [14] that coenzyme Q was essential to mitochondrial ATP forma-tion, i.e. to the most efficient mechanism which leads to the release of chemical energy housed in our nutrients. Several years later, Prof. P. Mitchell was awarded the Nobel Prize, for his studies centred on the vital role of coenzyme Q in oxidative phosphorylation. According to this early view, the quinone was considered as a substrate in excess concentration over the prosthetic groups in the lipoprotein com-plexes of the respiratory chain. The kinetic analyses of Kroger and Klingenberg [19] showed that steady-state respiration in submitochondrial particles could be repre-sented as a simple combination of two enzymes, the first one responsible for the reduction of coenzyme Q and the second one causing oxidation of ubiquinol. Experiments of direct titrations of CoQ-depleted mitochondria reconstituted with different CoQ supplements disclosed a Km of NADH oxidation close to a CoQ concentration of 4–10 mM in the lipid bilayer, whereas the Km for succinate oxida-tion was one order of magnitude lower [12]. The physiological concentration there-fore is not saturating, and even a small increase in the CoQ10 concentration of mitochondrial membranes could lead to an increased respiratory rate; on the other hand, even small decreases in cellular CoQ10 content may translate in remarkable impairment of mitochondrial functionality. The control exerted by CoQ concentra-tion over mitochondrial respiration could be of particular interest in situations of decreased CoQ levels and/or increased Km values for the quinone in some patho-logical states. In fact this observation could represent the biochemical mechanism by which exogenous coenzyme Q10 ameliorates the bioenergetic impairment in some mitochondrial myopathies and in cardiomyopathy [28, 31]. Modern views indicate that respiratory complexes may have a supramolecular organization, i.e. stable super complexes [13]. The advantage of this super complex organization would be a more efficient electron transfer by channelling of the redox intermedi-ates. Preliminary data suggest that alteration of the protein/phospholipid ratio and lipid peroxidation disaggregates the supercomplex organization with possible pathophysiological implications. Lenaz postulates [13] that in ageing, and in ischemic diseases, reactive oxygen species (ROS) produced by the mitochondrial respiratory chain induce a progressive peroxidation of mitochondrial phospholipids. This could lead to a dissociation of complex I–III aggregates and subsequent loss of facilitated electron channelling. Also according to this model, an increased concentration of coenzyme Q may, at least partially, counteract this deleterious effect of supercomplex disaggregation.

CoQ as an Antioxidant In its reduced form (ubiquinol), coenzyme Q acts as a phenolic antioxidant, undergoing hydrogen abstraction by free radicals; therefore, it acts like a chain-breaking antioxidant. This evidence has been produced by numerous experimental models, both in vivo and in vitro, using artificial membranes, isolated subcellular organelles, cultured cells, isolated perfused organs and clinical models. Lars Ernster, a pioneer of the studies on the location and the function of coenzyme Q in mitochondrial membranes, reviewed the mechanisms by which coenzyme Q, mainly in its reduced form, is currently believed to exert its antioxidant effect [11]. Experimental data strongly indicate that the intervention of coenzyme Q, in its reduced form, can be considered within the antioxidant preventive mechanisms. CoQH2 would reduce the perferryl species ($Fe^{+++} - O2^{\cdot-}$), thus preventing the radical attack that this species would initiate on fatty acids. By this mechanism, QH2 would practically prevent the formation of alkyl radicals (L•) and peroxyl radicals (LOO•). Ubiquinol may also act by slowing down the chain propagation reaction, according to the general mechanism of hydrogen donation to the radicals. Another mechanism by which ubiquinol exerts its antioxidant properties is the one explored by Packer, Kagan, et al. [17]. These authors demonstrated that reduced coenzyme Q regenerates α-tocopherol, the active form of vitamin E, by reducing the α-tocopherol radical. In these reactions, the ubisemiquinone radical is formed, whose presence in the mitochondrial respiratory chain has been known for the past 20 years. Ubisemiquinone is stabilized through the binding to special Q proteins. The presence of SOD and catalase would keep under control $O_2^{\cdot-}$ and the H_2O_2 arising from the autoxidation of the ubisemiquinone; however, it is unlikely that autoxidation of the ubisemiquinone species generates $O_2^{\cdot-}$ in the phospholipid environment. Ernster stresses the fact that coenzyme Q is the only a lipid-soluble antioxidant that animal cells can biosynthesize de novo and for which appropriate enzymatic mechanisms exist to regenerate the reduced form. We have demonstrated that reduced coenzyme Q exerts its antioxidant properties also by inactivating ferrimyoglobin, a species capable of triggering the oxidative attack at muscular and cardiac level [27]. Oxidative stress can of course attack the plasma membrane, which delimits the cell environment and also constitutes a protection against different kinds of oxidative insult from the environment. Different antioxidants are responsible for this protection, in particular ascorbate on the hydrophilic cell surface and CoQ, together with α-tocopherol in the hydrophobic phospholipid bilayer. In order to act as an antioxidant, CoQ must be in the reduced state; several enzymes exert this function of CoQ reductases. NADH-cytochrome *b5* reductase and NQO1 are among the principal reductase systems [32]. Numerous data indicate that the plasma membrane redox system plays an important role in preserving the antioxidant capacity during oxidative stress insults related both to the diet and to the ageing process. It is known that caloric restriction (CR) can attenuate oxidative stress and age-related oxidative stress. Plasma membrane redox system, of which CoQ is an essential constituent, is influenced by CR also through CoQ intervention. It was found that CoQ-dependent NADPH dehydrogenases were increate in plasma membranes from aged rats treated with caloric restriction [10]. As a consequence, the liver plasma membranes of aged rats treated with CR were more resistant to oxidative stress-induced lipid peroxidation compared to the membranes from rats fed ad libitum. Therefore, the antioxidant system in the plasma membrane is involved in the healthy ageing induced by CR. Also the plasma membrane content of CoQ, which declines with age, is enhanced by CR [32].

2.3   Endogenous and Nutritional Sources of Coenzyme Q10

Coenzyme Q10 is widely diffused in nature; thus, it is present in many vegetal and animal tissues which are part of our normal diet. Coenzyme Q10 is also actively synthesized by our cells. This is the reason it is not a vitamin according to the classical definition. So, our tissue levels of CoQ10 depend both on an endogenous biosynthesis and on an exogenous supply. Metabolic demand and the turnover rate of CoQ10 should also be taken into consideration when trying to establish a "nutritional status" of CoQ10. Nutritional intake: the content in CoQ9 and CoQ10 of different types of food was evaluated in a paper by [18]. CoQ9 is usually present in cereals, while CoQ10 is the ubiquinone of soybeans. CoQ10 is also present in walnuts, almonds, oils, fruits rich in oil and green vegetables; spinach is particularly rich in CoQ10. Some kinds of fish also have comparatively high amounts of CoQ10. On a weight basis, sardines have more than twice as much CoQ10 as beef; 1.6 kg of sardines contain 100 mg of CoQ10. Milk and cheese have a lower content of coenzyme Q10. It is difficult to assess the relative importance of endogenous biosynthesis and exogenous intake; the latter plays a significant role as well. Data from Kishi et al. (1986) showed that in patients under total parenteral nutrition (TPN), plasma levels of CoQ10 undergo a remarkable reduction (50 %) in just 1 week. This finding might be related to non-consumption of CoQ10 and/or its precursors present in the diet or to stressors that resulted in the patient requiring TPN. In our lab we often found plasma levels of CoQ10 close to or even lower than 0.1 µg/ml in traumatized patients. It is difficult to evaluate to what extent those data were related to TPN or to the serious clinical conditions of shocked patients. 0.1 µg/ml represents a very low value in as much as normal plasma levels are around 0.79 ± 0.2 µg/ml. Blood CoQ10 is mainly transported by LDL, although it is also present in the other classes of lipoproteins and in blood cells [49]. Its concentration is usually reported in micrograms/litre of plasma or micromoles/litre. But it is worthwhile to normalize these values according to the blood LDL content or at least to plasma cholesterol levels. The CoQ10/total cholesterol level could have a predictive value in cardiovascular disease as discussed below.

The endogenous synthesis of the quinone moiety of CoQ10 in our organism starts from phenylalanine or from tyrosine and the isoprenoid side chain derives from mevalonate. A series of vitamin cofactors is needed for this biosynthesis. It was highlighted that in a vitamin B6 deficiency plasma CoQ10 levels are also low and they increase upon improvement of the vitamin B6 deficiency status [55]. In eukaryotes the isoprenoid side chain of coenzyme Q is synthesized through the mevalonate pathway. Mevalonic acid (MVA) is converted to isopentenyl diphosphate (IPP). Dimethylallyl diphosphate acts as a primer and is progressively elongated by IPP to construct isoprenoid chains with progressively increasing length. Addition of a new isoprene to the growing polyisoprenoid chain can occur only at the alpha end since the process is energy requiring and there must be a leaving pyrophosphate group. Consequently, it is not possible to add a new isoprene to the omega end. During CoQ synthesis, solanesyl-PP or decaprenyl-PP is attached to the benzoquinone ring at the alpha end by the help of the leaving PP. The free end of the solanesol is the omega end without PP, and we do not know any enzymatic reaction which can mediate the addition of an additional isoprene. From a practical point of view, this implies that CoQ9, or a shorter homologue, taken with diet, cannot be elongated to CoQ10. As pointed out by [4, 5], dietary administration of CoQ9 or CoQ10 results in a number of metabolites which influence the endogenous synthesis of CoQ. In this respect, administration of CoQ9 may increase CoQ10 synthesis [4, 5].

Statins and CoQ10 Statins are 3-hydroxy-3-methylglutaryl coenzyme A (HMG-CoA) reductase inhibitors which decrease synthesis of mevalonate, a key metabolic step in the cholesterol synthesis pathway. These efficient drugs can produce a variety of muscle-related complaints or myopathies. Since the mevalonate pathway also leads to the biosynthesis of the isoprenoid side chain of coenzyme Q10, different studies have addressed the possibility of CoQ10 being an etiologic factor in statin myopathy. This issue has been extensively investigated, and it is worthwhile to mention two reviews by Littarru and Langsjoen [23, 24]. It was highlighted that, besides decreasing plasma CoQ10 levels, statin treatment also leads to lower lymphocyte levels of CoQ10. There are no univocal results about the effect of statin treatments on CoQ10 levels in skeletal muscle [21, 20], yet more recently [38] it was reported that high-dose statins did decrease muscle CoQ10 and mitochondrial respiratory chain activities, possibly related to reduction in the number or volume of muscle mitochondria. In a 2008 study, an inverse correlation between atorvastatin-induced changes in CoQ10 and BNP was found. It was concluded that long-term treatment with atorvastatin might increase plasma levels of BNP in patients with coronary heart disease when accompanied by a greater reduction in plasma CoQ10 [46]. Regarding the effect of CoQ10 supplementation, this was found not to improve statin tolerance or myalgia in one study [57], whereas [7] reported a positive effect of CoQ10 on pain severity and pain interference in daily activities in a group of statin-treated patients showing myopathic symptoms. A larger clinical trial where patients suffering from some statin side effects are treated with CoQ10 would shed more light on this issue.

Human CoQ10 Deficiencies Already in the past CoQ10 had been shown to be effective in a number of cases of mitochondrial myopathies, which were sometimes associated with low CoQ10 muscle levels. With the progress in molecular biology techniques, primary CoQ10 deficiencies, due to mutations in ubiquinone biosynthetic genes, have been identified, and they are associated with four major clinical phenotypes [39, 40]. Some of these syndromes have shown excellent responses to oral CoQ10 treatment. It has been ascertained that respiratory chain dysfunction and oxidative stress correlate with the severity of primary CoQ10 deficiency [39, 40]. Not all conditions respond to CoQ10 administration, perhaps also on the basis of the time when CoQ10 therapy was started; some of the responsive cases also showed an improvement of a nephropathy [26, 43].

2.4   Clinical Applications of Coenzyme Q10

In light of the mechanisms described above, a wide range of pathophysiological conditions associated with an increase in oxidative stress have been shown to be related to decreased CoQ levels and/or increased ubiquinone/total CoQ10 ratio. These conditions include physiological conditions such as the ageing process [37], intense physical exercise as well as a wide range of clinical conditions such as metabolic diseases, cardiovascular disease [22] and neurodegenerative and genetic disorders [34, 35, 50]. A detailed description of the role of CoQ10 in these conditions is beyond the scope of this review that will be limited to a brief description of the role of CoQ10 treatment in cardiovascular disease in light of its relevance and association with reproductive health and fertility issues [16, 36, 41].

In fact cardiovascular disease probably represents the clinical field where the beneficial role of CoQ10 has been better described, and its effects on CoQ10 can be ascribed to its bioenergetic role, to its capability of antagonizing oxidation of plasma LDL and to its effect in ameliorating endothelial function.

In this context, support of mitochondrial bioenergetics is directly linked to myocardial contractility, while the latter two mechanisms are associated to the systemic antioxidant protection exerted by CoQ in the vasculature that has also direct important implication in reproductive health.

It is currently believed that high levels of LDL, as well as smoking and hypertension, are primary risk factors, among those contributing to cardiovascular disease. Biochemical mechanisms responsible for the atherogenicity of LDL have been extensively addressed, and experimental evidence has been produced indicating that oxidatively modified LDL become atherogenic. It was found that endothelial cells are involved in the oxidative attack against LDL [10] as described above. Oxidative attack on LDL deeply affects the apoprotein moiety as well. As a consequence of these changes, LDL are no longer "recognized" by the normal receptors and are taken up more readily by the scavenger receptors of macrophages. LDL leave the blood stream, penetrate the endothelial cell lining and reach the subendothelial space, where they undergo oxidative attack. Oxidatively modified LDL are capable of triggering further events, including platelet activation, and exert a chemotactic attraction on circulating monocytes, which migrate to the subendothelial space, where they become macrophages. These cells have only low levels of the classical LDL receptor; nonetheless, they are able to take up more rapidly oxidatively modified LDL, and this uptake involves a different receptor, called the "scavenger receptor". As discussed above, oxidatively modified LDL are easily recognized by the scavenger receptors. These events lead to an accumulation of lipids, mainly cholesterol and cholesterol esters, in the macrophages, which will become lipid-laden foam cells. Foam cells may be considered the essence of the atheromatous lesions. LDL are endowed with a number of lipid-soluble antioxidants capable of preventing or minimizing lipid peroxidation.

Plasma levels of CoQ10 have been extensively investigated [52]. Most plasma CoQ10 is transported by LDL where, together with vitamin E, it exerts its antioxidant protection. As initially pointed out by Stocker [49], ubiquinol-10 is the most reactive antioxidant in LDL, and although it is present at lower concentrations compared to vitamin E, it is able to regenerate α-tocopherol from the tocopherol radical, making the vitamin E-ubiquinol duo the most important antioxidant system in LDL. CoQ10-enriched LDL, isolated from plasma of healthy volunteers orally treated with CoQ10 for a few days, were less susceptible to peroxidizability in vitro, compared to the same LDL in basal conditions [25]. Besides decreasing LDL peroxidizability, CoQ10 could have a direct antiatherosclerotic effect; in fact animal studies have shown that CoQ10 administration attenuates aortic atherosclerotic lesions [44, 56].

Besides LDL peroxidation, another early event in atherogenesis, also deeply associated with oxidative damage to the vasculature, is represented by an alteration of endothelial functionality that results in lowered nitric oxide (NO) bioavailability potentially coupled with noxious formation of peroxynitrate ultimately resulting in amplified oxidative stress, decreased flexibility of the arteries and enhanced platelet aggregation and endothelial adhesion, all mechanisms directly linked with atherosclerosis progression. In reproductive medicine this condition is associated also with erectile dysfunction, a condition often associated with vascular oxidative stress [30]. CoQ10 beneficial effects on endothelial functionality were first seen by Watts et al. in patients affected by type II diabetes [54] and then further explored by our group in patients affected by ischemic heart disease [2]. Among the recent data produced by our lab, CoQ10 was found to improve endothelium-bound extracellular SOD (ecSOD) [49] in patients affected by coronary artery disease (CAD). CAD patients have decreased levels of ecSOD, an enzyme which is thought to protect blood vessels against oxidant-induced damage. CoQ10 treatment determined a significant improvement in ecSOD activity, more pronounced in patients who had initial low values of ecSOD itself, therefore, likely exposed to greater oxidative stress. This effect was accompanied by an increase of maximal oxygen uptake and of flow-mediated dilation (FMD), a recognized index of endothelial function.

Clinical applications of CoQ10 in reproductive medicine will be extensively discussed in other chapters of this book. In summary the clinical applications show a beneficial effect of CoQ10 supplementation in mitigating oxidative stress in sperm cells and improve their functionality. Impairment of mitochondrial bioenergetics and oxidative stress are known to be involved in sperm motility. An update of CoQ10 implications in male infertility, covering also the early studies, was given by Mancini et al. [24]. Recent publication from our group confirmed, in a placebo-controlled double-blind randomized trial, the efficacy of CoQ10 treatment in improving semen quality in men with idiopathic infertility [1, 51]. Oxidized and reduced CoQ10 concentration significantly increased both in seminal plasma and sperm cells, together with sperm motility, after 6 months of therapy with 200 mg/day CoQ10. The increased concentration of CoQ10 and QH2 (reduced CoQ10) in seminal plasma and sperm cells, the improvement of semen kinetic features and treatment and the evidence of a direct correlation between CoQ10 concentrations and sperm motility strongly support a cause-effect relationship. Similar results were found by Safarinejad [42]. In this study 212 infertile men with idiopathic oligoasthenoteratospermia were treated with 300 mg/day CoQ10 or placebo for 26 weeks. Statistically significant improvement was found, in the CoQ10 group, regarding sperm count and motility values, with a positive correlation between treatment duration of CoQ10 and sperm count as well as mean sperm motility. The CoQ10 group had a significant decrease in serum FSH and LH at the 26-week treatment phase. The authors highlight that a lower serum FSH implies a better spermatogenesis. Moreover, inhibin B, which reflects Sertoli cell function, increased in the CoQ10 group.

In the field of reproductive medicine, CoQ10 has been also linked to folliculogenesis in the female and embryo parameters relevant to in vitro fertilization embryo transfer [6]. A study from Stojkovic et al. [45] has looked into the effect of CoQ10 as a supplement for the in vitro culture of bovine embryos and found a significantly higher rate of early embryo cleavage, blastocyst formation rate, hatching rate, percentage of expanding blastocysts and a larger size of the inner cell mass (ICM). In the same paper, the authors observed an increased ATP content in the group of embryos cultured with CoQ10. All of those parameters suggest improved embryo quality.

In a recent paper, we evaluated CoQ10 content in human follicular fluid in relation to oocyte fertilization and embryo grading [53]. CoQ10 levels resulted significantly higher in mature versus dysmorphic oocytes. Similarly, levels resulted significantly enhanced in grading I–II versus grading III–IV embryos. This data could highlight a role of CoQ10 in protecting follicular lipoproteins from oxidation, preserving their functionality. Moreover, CoQ10 might act in lowering mitochondrial dysfunction in granulosa cells due to its bioenergetic involvement. Finally CoQ10 has been shown to have an important effect also during pregnancy: Teran et al. [47] reported the results of a CoQ10 supplementation in reducing the risk of preeclampsia. Pregnant women at increased risk of preeclampsia either received 200 mg of CoQ10 or placebo daily from 20 weeks of pregnancy until delivery. The overall rate of preeclampsia was 20 %, and there was a significant difference in the placebo group (25.6 %) compared to the CoQ10-treated one (14.4 %). Preeclampsia is a common disorder of human pregnancy in which the normal haemodynamic response to pregnancy is compromised. It remains a leading cause of maternal morbidity and mortality and is associated with a significant increase in perinatal mortality. The newly recognized role of CoQ10 in improving endothelial function [49] could have a particular importance in preeclampsia in which endothelial dysfunction is known to play a pathogenetic role [48].

References

1. Balercia G, Buldreghini E, Vignini A, Tiano L, Paggi F, Amoroso S, Ricciardo-Lamonica G, Boscaro M, Lenzi A, Littarru G. Coenzyme Q10 treatment in infertile men with idiopathic asthenozoospermia: a placebo-controlled, double-blind randomized trial. Fertil Steril. 2009;91(5):1785–92. doi:10.1016/j.fertnstert.2008.02.119.
2. Belardinelli R, Muçaj A, Lacalaprice F, Solenghi M, Seddaiu G, Principi F, Tiano L, Littarru GP. Coenzyme Q10 and exercise training in chronic heart failure. Eur Heart J. 2006; 27(22):2675–81.
3. Bentinger M, Tekle M, Brismar K, Chojnacki T, Swiezewska E, Dallner G. Polyisoprenoid epoxides stimulate the biosynthesis of coenzyme Q and inhibit cholesterol synthesis. J Biol Chem. 2008a;283(21):14645–53. doi:10.1074/jbc.M710202200.
4. Bentinger M, Tekle M, Brismar K, Chojnacki T, Swiezewska E, Dallner G. Stimulation of coenzyme Q synthesis. Biofactors. 2008b;32(1–4):99–111.
5. Bentov Y, Casper RF. The aging oocyte--can mitochondrial function be improved? Fertil Steril. 2013;99(1):18–22. doi:10.1016/j.fertnstert.2012.11.031apr.
6. Caso G, Kelly P, McNurlan MA, Lawson WE. Effect of coenzyme q10 on myopathic symptoms in patients treated with statins. Am J Cardiol. 2007;99(10):1409–12.
7. Crane FL, Hatefi Y, Lester RL, Widmer C. Isolation of a quinone from beef heart mitochondria. Biochim Biophys Acta. 1957;25(1):220–1.
8. Dallner G, Stocker R. Encyclopedia of dietary supplements. New York: Marcel Dekker; 2005. p. 121.
9. De Cabo R, Cabello R, Rios M, López-Lluch G, Ingram DK, Lane MA, Navas P. Calorie restriction attenuates age-related alterations in the plasma membrane antioxidant system in rat liver. Exp Gerontol. 2004;39(3):297–304.
10. Ernster L, Forsmark-Andrée P. Ubiquinol: an endogenous antioxidant in aerobic organisms. Clin Investig. 1993;71(8 Suppl):S60–5. PubMed PMID: 8241707.
11. Estornell E, Fato R, Castelluccio C, Cavazzoni M, Parenti Castelli G, Lenaz G. Saturation kinetics of coenzyme Q in NADH and succinate oxidation in beef heart mitochondria. FEBS Lett. 1992;311(2):107–9. PubMed PMID: 1327877.
12. Genova ML, Bianchi C, Lenaz G. Supercomplex organization of the mitochondrial respiratory chain and the role of the Coenzyme Q pool: pathophysiological implications. Biofactors. 2005;25(1–4):5–20.
13. Green DE, Tzagoloff A. The mitochondrial electron transfer chain. Arch Biochem Biophys. 1966;116(1):293–304. PubMed PMID: 4289862.
14. Groneberg DA, Kindermann B, Althammer M, Klapper M, Vormann J, Littarru GP, Döring F. Coenzyme Q10 affects expression of genes involved in cell signalling, metabolism and transport in human CaCo-2 cells. Int J Biochem Cell Biol. 2005;37(6):1208–18. 9
15. Heida KY, Bots ML, de Groot CJ, van Dunné FM, Hammoud NM, Hoek A, Laven JS, Maas AH, Roeters van Lennep JE, Velthuis BK, Franx A. Cardiovascular risk management after reproductive and pregnancy-related disorders: a Dutch multidisciplinary evidence-based guideline. Eur J Prev Cardiol. 2016. pii: 2047487316659573. [Epub ahead of print] Review.
16. Kagan V, Serbinova E, Packer L. Antioxidant effects of ubiquinones in microsomes and mitochondria are mediated by tocopherol recycling. Biochem Biophys Res Commun. 1990;169(3): 851–7. PubMed PMID: 2114108.
17. Kamei M, Fujita T, Kanbe T, Sasaki K, Oshiba K, Otani S, Matsui-Yuasa I, Morisawa S. The distribution and content of ubiquinone in foods. Int J Vitam Nutr Res. 1986;56(1):57–63. PubMed PMID: 3710719.

18. Kröger A, Klingenberg M. Eur J Biochem. 1973;34:358.
19. Laaksonen R, Jokelainen K, Sahi T, Tikkanen MJ, Himberg JJ. Decreases in serum ubiquinone concentrations do not result in reduced levels in muscle tissue during short-term simvastatin treatment in humans. Clin Pharmacol Ther. 1995;57(1):62–6. PubMed PMID: 7828383.
20. Lamperti C, Naini AB, Lucchini V, Prelle A, Bresolin N, Moggio M, Sciacco M, Kaufmann P, DiMauro S. Muscle coenzyme Q10 level in statin-related myopathy. Arch Neurol. 2005; 62(11):1709–12.
21. Littarru GP, Tiano L, Belardinelli R, Watts GF. Coenzyme Q(10), endothelial function, and cardiovascular disease. Biofactors. 2011;37(5):366–73. doi:10.1002/biof.154.
22. Littarru GP, Langsjoen P. Coenzyme Q10 and statins: biochemical and clinical implications. Mitochondrion. 2007;7 Suppl:S168–74. 7
23. Mancini A, De Marinis L, Littarru GP, Balercia G. An update of Coenzyme Q10 implications in male infertility: biochemical and therapeutic aspects. Biofactors. 2005;25(1–4):165–74.
24. Marcoff L, Thompson PD. The role of coenzyme Q10 in statin-associated myopathy: a systematic review. J Am Coll Cardiol. 2007;12;49(23):2231–7. Review. PubMed PMID: 17560286.
25. Mohr D, Bowry VW, Stocker R. Dietary supplementation with coenzyme Q10 results in increased levels of ubiquinol-10 within circulating lipoproteins and increased resistance of human low-density lipoprotein to the initiation of lipid peroxidation. Biochim Biophys Acta. 1992;1126(3):247–54. PubMed PMID: 1637852.
26. Montini G, Malaventura C, Salviati L. Early coenzyme Q10 supplementation in primary coenzyme Q10 deficiency. N Engl J Med. 2008;358(26):2849–50. doi:10.1056/NEJMc0800582.
27. Mordente A, Martorana GE, Santini SA, Miggiano GA, Petitti T, Giardina B, Battino M, Littarru GP. Antioxidant effect of coenzyme Q on hydrogen peroxide-activated myoglobin. Clin Investig. 1993;71(8 Suppl):S92–6. PubMed PMID: 8241712.
28. Mortensen SA, Rosenfeldt F, Kumar A, Dolliner P, Filipiak KJ, Pella D, Alehagen U, Steurer G, GP L, Q-SYMBIO Study Investigators. The effect of coenzyme Q10 on morbidity and mortality in chronic heart failure: results from Q-SYMBIO: a randomized double-blind trial. JACC Heart Fail. 2014;2(6):641–9. doi:10.1016/j.jchf.2014.06.008.
29. Morton RA. Ubiquinone Nature. 1958;182(4652):1764–7.
30. Musicki B, Bella AJ, Bivalacqua TJ, Davies KP, DiSanto ME, Gonzalez-Cadavid NF, Hannan JL, Kim NN, Podlasek CA, Wingard CJ, Burnett AL. Basic science evidence for the link between erectile dysfunction and cardiometabolic dysfunction. J Sex Med. 2015;12(12):2233–55. doi:10.1111/jsm.13069. PubMed PMID: 26646025; PubMed Central PMCID: PMC4854187.
31. Naini A, Lewis VJ, Hirano M, DiMauro S. Primary coenzyme Q10 deficiency and the brain. Biofactors. 2003;18(1–4):145–52.
32. Navas P, Villalba JM, de Cabo R. The importance of plasma membrane coenzyme Q in aging and stress responses. Mitochondrion. 2007;7(Suppl):S34–40.
33. Pagano G, Aiello Talamanca A, Castello G, Cordero MD, d'Ischia M, Gadaleta MN, Pallardó FV, Petrović S, Tiano L, Zatterale A. Current experience in testing mitochondrial nutrients in disorders featuring oxidative stress and mitochondrial dysfunction: rational design of chemoprevention trials. Int J Mol Sci. 2014a;15(11):20169–208. doi:10.3390/ijms151120169. PubMed PMID: 25380523; PubMed Central PMCID: PMC4264162.
34. Pagano G, Talamanca AA, Castello G, Cordero MD, d'Ischia M, Gadaleta MN, Pallardó FV, Petrović S, Tiano L, Zatterale A. Oxidative stress and mitochondrial dysfunction across broad-ranging pathologies: toward mitochondria-targeted clinical strategies. Oxidative Med Cell Longev. 2014b;2014:541230. doi:10.1155/2014/541230. PubMed PMID: 24876913; PubMed Central PMCID: PMC4024404.
35. Perry JR, Murray A, Day FR, Ong KK. Molecular insights into the aetiology of female reproductive ageing. Nat Rev Endocrinol. 2015;11(12):725–34. doi:10.1038/nrendo.2015.167.
36. Phillipson OT. Management of the aging risk factor for Parkinson's disease. Neurobiol Aging. 2014;35(4):847–57. doi:10.1016/j.neurobiolaging.2013.10.073.

37. Päivä H, Thelen KM, Van Coster R, Smet J, De Paepe B, Mattila KM, Laakso J, Lehtimäki T, von Bergmann K, Lütjohann D, Laaksonen R. High-dose statins and skeletal muscle metabolism in humans: a randomized, controlled trial. Clin Pharmacol Ther. 2005;78(1):60–8.
38. Quinzii CM, López LC, Von-Moltke J, Naini A, Krishna S, Schuelke M, Salviati L, Navas P, DiMauro S, Hirano M. Respiratory chain dysfunction and oxidative stress correlate with severity of primary CoQ10 deficiency. FASEB J. 2008b;22(6):1874–85. doi:10.1096/fj.07-100149. PubMed PMID: 18230681; PubMed Central PMCID: PMC2731482.
39. Quinzii CM, López LC, Naini A, DiMauro S, Hirano M. Human CoQ10 deficiencies. Biofactors. 2008a;32(1–4):113–8. PubMed PMID: 19096106; PubMed Central PMCID: PMC3625975.
40. Roberts JM, Mascalzoni D, Ness RB, Poston L, Global Pregnancy Collaboration. Collaboration to understand complex diseases: preeclampsia and adverse pregnancy outcomes. Hypertension. 2016;67(4):681–7. doi:10.1161/HYPERTENSIONAHA.115.06133.
41. Safarinejad MR. Efficacy of coenzyme Q10 on semen parameters, sperm function and reproductive hormones in infertile men. J Urol. 2009;182(1):237–48. doi:10.1016/j.juro.2009.02.121.
42. Salviati L, Sacconi S, Murer L, Zacchello G, Franceschini L, Laverda AM, Basso G, Quinzii C, Angelini C, Hirano M, Naini AB, Navas P, DiMauro S, Montini G. Infantile encephalomyopathy and nephropathy with CoQ10 deficiency: a CoQ10-responsive condition. Neurology. 2005;65(4):606–8.
43. Singh RB, Shinde SN, Chopra RK, Niaz MA, Thakur AS, Onouchi Z. Effect of coenzyme Q10 on experimental atherosclerosis and chemical composition and quality of atheroma in rabbits. Atherosclerosis. 2000;148(2):275–82.
44. Stojkovic M, Westesen K, Zakhartchenko V, Stojkovic P, Boxhammer K, Wolf E. Coenzyme Q(10) in submicron-sized dispersion improves development, hatching, cell proliferation, and adenosine triphosphate content of in vitro-produced bovine embryos. Biol Reprod. 1999; 61(2):541–7.
45. Suzuki T, Nozawa T, Sobajima M, Igarashi N, Matsuki A, Fujii N, Inoue H. Atorvastatin-induced changes in plasma coenzyme q10 and brain natriuretic peptide in patients with coronary artery disease. Int Heart J. 2008;49(4):423–33.
46. Teran E, Hernandez I, Nieto B, Tavara R, Ocampo JE, Calle A. Coenzyme Q10 supplementation during pregnancy reduces the risk of pre-eclampsia. Int J Gynaecol Obstet. 2009;105(1):43–5. doi:10.1016/j.ijgo.2008.11.033.
47. Teran E, Escudero C, Vivero S, Molina G, Calle A. NO in early pregnancy and development of preeclampsia. Hypertension. 2006;47(4):e17. 3
48. Thomas SR, Witting PK, Stocker R. A role for reduced coenzyme Q in atherosclerosis? Biofactors. 1999;9(2–4):207–24.
49. Tiano L, Belardinelli R, Carnevali P, Principi F, Seddaiu G, Littarru GP. Effect of coenzyme Q10 administration on endothelial function and extracellular superoxide dismutase in patients with ischaemic heart disease: a double-blind, randomized controlled study. Eur Heart J. 2007;28(18):2249–55. PubMed PMID:17644511.
50. Tiano L, Busciglio J. Mitochondrial dysfunction and Down's syndrome: is there a role for coenzyme Q(10) ? Biofactors. 2011;37(5):386–92. doi:10.1002/biof.184.
51. Tirabassi G, Vignini A, Tiano L, Buldreghini E, Brugè F, Silvestri S, Orlando P, D'Aniello A, Mazzanti L, Lenzi A, Balercia G. Protective effects of coenzyme Q10 and aspartic acid on oxidative stress and DNA damage in subjects affected by idiopathic asthenozoospermia. Endocrine. 2015;49(2):549–52. doi:10.1007/s12020-014-0432-6.
52. Tomasetti M, Alleva R, Solenghi MD, Littarru GP. Distribution of antioxidants among blood components and lipoproteins: significance of lipids/CoQ10 ratio as a possible marker of increased risk for atherosclerosis. Biofactors. 1999;9(2–4):231–40.
53. Turi A, Giannubilo SR, Brugè F, Principi F, Battistoni S, Santoni F, Tranquilli AL, Littarru G, Tiano L. Coenzyme Q10 content in follicular fluid and its relationship with oocyte fertilization and embryo grading. Arch Gynecol Obstet. 2012;285(4):1173–6. doi:10.1007/s00404-011-2169-2.

54. Watts GF, Playford DA, Croft KD, Ward NC, Mori TA, Burke V. Coenzyme Q(10) improves endothelial dysfunction of the brachial artery in Type II diabetes mellitus. Diabetologia. 2002;45(3):420–6.
55. Willis R, Anthony M, Sun L, Honse Y, Qiao G. Clinical implications of the correlation between coenzyme Q10 and vitamin B6 status. Biofactors. 1999;9(2–4):359–63.
56. Witting PK, Pettersson K, Letters J, Stocker R. Anti-atherogenic effect of coenzyme Q10 in apolipoprotein E gene knockout mice. Free Radic Biol Med. 2000;29(3–4):295–305.
57. Young JM, Florkowski CM, Molyneux SL, McEwan RG, Frampton CM, George PM, Scott RS. Effect of coenzyme Q(10) supplementation on simvastatin-induced myalgia. Am J Cardiol. 2007;100(9):1400–3.

Carnitine in Male Infertility

3

Andrea Sansone, Loredana Gandini, Francesco Lombardo, and Andrea Lenzi

3.1 Carnitine: An Introduction

Carnitine is an amino acid derivative, mainly obtained through alimentary intake although its synthesis is possible in men, acting as a cofactor in lipid processing in the mitochondria [13]. Carnitine is fundamental in energy production, as a substrate for beta-oxidation, and is also involved in the use of different substrates for energy production in the mitochondria (Fig. 3.1). Furthermore, carnitine plays a role in the removal of short and medium chain fatty acids accumulating in the mitochondria through metabolism [1]. In fact, energy regulation in response to endo- and extracellular and microenvironmental stimuli is mediated by the carnitine system. This system, which comprises L-carnitine, its derivatives, and the proteins involved in its transformation and transport, has a role both in energy metabolism in the cells and in protection against oxidation. The system also acts in peroxisomal lipid oxidation unrelated to energy production and in the acylation and deacylation of proteins in the endoplasmic reticulum, the exchange of membrane phospholipids, and the maintenance of cellular osmotic balance. These antioxidant properties help preventing membrane and DNA damage resulting from oxidative stress [3]. Male germ line cells have a low number of antioxidant molecules and enzymes due to their lack of cytoplasm and have a special polyunsaturated fatty acid (PUFA) structure in the membrane. PUFA are particularly susceptible to peroxidation phenomena associated with forms of oligoasthenoteratozoospermia (OAT). A crucial role for carnitine in male infertility has been postulated as the concentration of carnitine in the male genital tract, and particularly in the epididymis, is remarkably

A. Sansone • L. Gandini • F. Lombardo (✉) • A. Lenzi
Sapienza – University of Rome, Department of Experimental Medicine,
Section of Medical Pathophysiology, Food Science and Endocrinology,
Rome, Italy
e-mail: francesco.lombardo@uniroma1.it

© Springer International Publishing Switzerland 2017
G. Balercia et al. (eds.), *Antioxidants in Andrology*, Trends in Andrology and Sexual Medicine, DOI 10.1007/978-3-319-41749-3_3

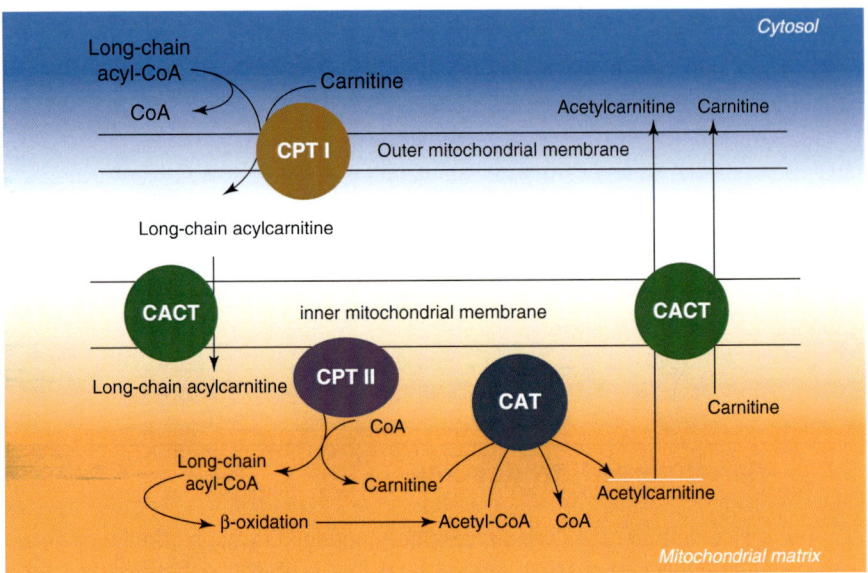

Fig. 3.1 The mitochondrial carnitine system. *CoA* coenzyme A, *CAT* carnitine acetyltransferase, *CPT I* carnitine palmitoyltransferase I, *CPT II* carnitine palmitoyltransferase II, *CACT* carnitine-acylcarnitine translocase

high [12]. Carnitine may in fact act as a scavenging mechanism for reactive oxygen species (ROS) in the prevention of some forms of idiopathic male infertility. The efficacy of the use of various antioxidants as a therapeutic tool has been demonstrated in various controlled studies on selected caseloads of infertile subjects [16]. There is ample experimental evidence to suggest that carnitine has a protective role against oxidative stress [16]. The mechanism through which it expresses its antioxidant properties is not yet completely clear, although there is considerable evidence that its main protective action is in the membrane systems. Despite lacking the typical features of an antioxidant compound, such as electron releasing groups, carnitine and some of its short-chain derivatives (including acetyl L-carnitine [ALC] and propyl L-carnitine) can reduce lipid peroxidation processes in the cell membrane following oxidative stress. Given these features, these molecules may be particularly useful in conditions affecting organs and tissues with highly active lipid metabolism, such as the epididymis. The effect on biological membranes is critically involved in protection of cell structure and prevention of cell death by apoptosis. Carnitine – in the form of short-chain esters – has been observed in the double lipid layer of the biological membranes near the glycerol skeleton, affecting its fluidity and inhibiting lipid peroxidation [14]. In the mitochondrial membrane, carnitine provides protection against oxidation and by scavenging free radicals (of which the mitochondrion is a source) reduces emission of calcium ions. Carnitine was also proven able to prevent FAS/FAS ligand-induced apoptosis and activation of recombinant caspases 3, 7, and 8 [17, 19].

3.2 Carnitine in Male Infertility

The presence of an active lipid metabolism, a high concentration of PUFA in the sperm membranes, and a significant concentration of unsaturated fatty acids in the seminal plasma clearly show the role of lipids as an important energy reserve and essential structural and metabolic element for the spermatozoa. These also make good targets for the action of carnitine and its derivatives, whose concentrations in the epididymis and seminal plasma, as previously stated, are tens of times higher than in any other area of the body.

3.2.1 In Vivo Effects of Carnitine Administration

These actions all support the use of carnitine as a possible therapy for selected forms of male infertility, and it has already been proposed for the treatment of conditions involving altered semen parameters [1, 11, 13]. However, the validity of most preliminary studies investigating the role of carnitine administration on male fertility has been questioned, as the lack of a control group made results unreliable.

Since then, several randomized controlled trials assessing the effects of carnitine administration on semen parameters have been published [4, 9, 13, 15, 21]. To the present date, most studies have shown some degree of improvements in subjects undergoing treatment with carnitine, either alone or together with other antioxidants (Table 3.1). However, not all subjects respond equally to treatment: the rationale for the lack of response lies in the baseline conditions of the patient undergoing therapy. Male genital tract infections, including epididymitis, are associated with a marked decrease in seminal plasma carnitine concentration. In these patients, administration of carnitine alone might not have the desired effects, as the antioxidant effects of the treatment might not be enough to prevent further inflammation-related oxidative stress. Therefore, antibiotic treatment should be suggested before administering carnitine [17], as this would improve chances at obtaining better semen parameters. On the other hand, lipid peroxidation might persist despite antibiotic treatment, and patients with leukocytospermia are less prone to respond to treatment with combined L-carnitine and acetyl-L-carnitine despite being asymptomatic [22, 23]. In these subjects, improvements have been reported in terms of vitality only, despite an increase in motility and viability in non-leukocytospermic men.

Combined treatment was also effective in increasing semen quality in selected populations, particularly in groups with worse baseline conditions [13, 15]. This might reflect underlying conditions, including excessive ROS generation, which might be treated by administration of carnitine and its derivatives. Carnitine and acetyl-L-carnitine were administered together with cinnoxicam, a nonsteroidal anti-inflammatory drug, in an experimental study aimed to assess the possible effects of these drugs on male fertility. In both idiopathic and varicocele-associated OAT, despite some negligible side effects, the therapy resulted significantly more effective than L-carnitine/acetyl-L-carnitine alone or than placebo in terms of

Table 3.1 In vivo studies on the effects of carnitine

Reference	Study type	Patients	Intervention	Results
[22]	Open trial	54 men with PVE, with or without leukocytospermia	L-carnitine 2 g/day + LAC 1 g/day for 3 months	Increased sperm motility and viability in men without leukocytospermia
Vicari et al. [23]	Open trial	98 men with leukocytospermia and PVE	Carnitines and/or NSAIDs for 2–4 months	Increased sperm motility and viability in patients pretreated with NSAIDs
Lenzi et al. [13]	RCT	100 OAT men	L-carnitine 2 g/day for 2 months	Improved sperm motility, concentration and linearity
Lenzi et al. [15]	RCT	60 OAT men	L-carnitine 2 g/day + LAC 1 g/day for 6 months	Improved sperm motility
Cavallini et al. [7]	RCT	380 OAT men	L-carnitine 2 g/day + LAC 1 g/day, with or without Cinnoxicam 30 mg every 4 days, for 6 months	Increased sperm concentration, motility, and morphology in patients with grade I-IV varicocele
Garolla et al. [9]	RCT	30 asthenozoospermic men	L-carnitine 2 g/day for 3 months	Improved sperm motility only in patients with normal levels of PHGPx
Balercia et al. [4]	RCT	60 OAT men	L-carnitine 3 g/day, LAC 3 g/day, or L-carnitine 2 g/day + LAC 1 g/day for 6 months	Improved sperm motility and velocity
Sigman et al. [21]	RCT	21 asthenozoospermic men	L-carnitine 2 g/day + LAC 1 g/day for 6 months	No effects on sperm motility or total motile sperm counts
Moradi et al. [18]	RCT	52 men with idiopathic infertility	Either L-carnitine 25 mg/day or clomiphene citrate 2 g/day for 3 months	Improved seminal volume, sperm concentration and motility
Busetto et al. [6]	Open trial	114 astenoteratozoospermic men	Proxeed 1/day for 4 months	Increased sperm motility

Abbreviations: RCT randomized control trial, *OAT* oligoasthenoteratozoospermia, *PVE* prostatovesiculoepididymitis, *LAC* L-acetyl-carnitine, *NSAIDs* nonsteroidal anti-inflammatory drugs, *PHGPx* phospholipid hydroperoxide glutathione peroxidase improvements of sperm concentration, motility, and morphology [7]. Motility seems to be the parameter most frequently improved following administration of carnitine. This has been confirmed even in association with other compounds with antioxidant properties [6], although the association of carnitine and clomiphene citrate resulted in significantly increased sperm motility and concentration [18], suggesting a possible use as a first-line treatment for idiopathic OAT.

3.2.2 Carnitine Administration and Assisted Reproduction Techniques

In assisted reproduction techniques (ART), obtaining sperm of the highest quality is of the utmost importance in order to provide the best chances at fecundation. Spermatozoa obtained through testicular extraction often demonstrate poor quality and nonprogressive movement, and therefore in vitro culture is required in order to obtain viable sperm cells. Because of its effects on oxidative stress and energy production, L-carnitine has also been used in vitro in ART as a tool for improving semen quality. Supplementation of L-carnitine and acetyl-L-carnitine to the culture medium was able to reduce in vitro oxidative stress, improving motility and chromatin quality [2] in rodent models. In men, administration of L-carnitine to the culture medium was found to be toxic for spermatozoa at higher concentrations ($\geq$ 50 mg/ml) while, at the same time, able to improve motility at lower concentration (0.5 mg/ml), with no effects on DNA oxidation and viability [5].

Administration of oral supplements of L-carnitine and acetyl-L-carnitine has also been suggested as a treatment for OAT men who are about to start semen collection for ART. Improvements in conventional parameters have been observed in treated subjects, as previously stated, but a statistically significant reduction in nuclear fragmentation and increase in sperm viability has also been observed in subjects undergoing treatment with L-carnitine and acetyl-L-carnitine compared to placebo. Unexpectedly, increased pregnancy rate and embryo quality have also been described in treated subjects. Whether the existence of markers predicting a positive response to treatment is a topic open for debate, but to the present date, best results have been observed in subjects with severe OAT. Evidence in support of this treatment is still far from conclusive, but it's clearly possible that subjects undergoing treatment might benefit from treatment even when natural fertilization fails.

3.2.3 Safety Concerns for Carnitine

Safety assessment is a recurring issue for many of the nutritional supplements administered for the most different conditions. While some studies suggest that oral intake of these compounds is safe and free from side effects, there have been cases of reported liver toxicity in subjects undergoing treatment with different nutritional supplements [8, 20].

To the present date, oral intake of carnitine and acetyl-L-carnitine has not been associated with severe side effects. Some authors have reported unpleasant body odor, flatulence, and increased appetite in subjects taking excessive dosages (ranging between 3000 and 7000 mg daily). No significant side effects were reported with 2000 mg/day or less, proving that carnitine administration is safe for its use in treatment of idiopathic male infertility [10].

References

1. Agarwal A, Said TM. Carnitines and male infertility. Reprod Biomed Online. 2004;8(4): 376–84.
2. Aliabadi E, Soleimani Mehranjani M, Borzoei Z, Talaei-Khozani T, Mirkhani H, Tabesh H. Effects of L-carnitine and L-acetyl-carnitine on testicular sperm motility and chromatin quality. Iranian J Reprod Med. 2012;10(2):77–82.
3. Arduini A. Carnitine and its acyl esters as secondary antioxidants? Am Heart J. 1992;123(6): 1726–7.
4. Balercia G, Regoli F, Armeni T, Koverech A, Mantero F, Boscaro M. Placebo-controlled double-blind randomized trial on the use of L-carnitine, L-acetylcarnitine, or combined L-carnitine and L-acetylcarnitine in men with idiopathic asthenozoospermia. Fertil Steril. 2005;84(3):662–71. doi:10.1016/j.fertnstert.2005.03.064.
5. Banihani S, Sharma R, Bayachou M, Sabanegh E, Agarwal A. Human sperm DNA oxidation, motility and viability in the presence of L-carnitine during in vitro incubation and centrifugation. Andrologia. 2012;44(Suppl 1):505–12. doi:10.1111/j.1439-0272.2011.01216.x.
6. Busetto GM, Koverech A, Messano M, Antonini G, De Berardinis E, Gentile V. Prospective open-label study on the efficacy and tolerability of a combination of nutritional supplements in primary infertile patients with idiopathic astenoteratozoospermia. Arch Ital Urol Androl. 2012;84(3):137–40.
7. Cavallini G, Ferraretti AP, Gianaroli L, Biagiotti G, Vitali G. Cinnoxicam and L-carnitine/acetyl-L-carnitine treatment for idiopathic and varicocele-associated oligoasthenospermia. J Androl. 2004;25(5):761–70. discussion 71-2
8. Garcia-Cortes M, Robles-Diaz M, Ortega-Alonso A, Medina-Caliz I, Andrade RJ. Hepatotoxicity by dietary supplements: a tabular listing and clinical characteristics. Int J Mol Sci. 2016;17(4):537. doi:10.3390/ijms17040537.
9. Garolla A, Maiorino M, Roverato A, Roveri A, Ursini F, Foresta C. Oral carnitine supplementation increases sperm motility in asthenozoospermic men with normal sperm phospholipid hydroperoxide glutathione peroxidase levels. Fertil Steril. 2005;83(2):355–61. doi:10.1016/j.fertnstert.2004.10.010.
10. Hathcock JN, Shao A. Risk assessment for carnitine. Regul Toxicol Pharmacol. 2006;46(1):23–8. doi:10.1016/j.yrtph.2006.06.007.
11. Isidori AM, Pozza C, Gianfrilli D, Isidori A. Medical treatment to improve sperm quality. Reprod Biomed Online. 2006;12(6):704–14.
12. Lenzi A, Lombardo F, Gandini L, Dondero F. Metabolism and action of L-carnitine: its possible role in sperm tail function. Arch Ital Urol Nefrol Androl. 1992;64(2):187–96.
13. Lenzi A, Lombardo F, Sgro P, Salacone P, Caponecchia L, Dondero F, et al. Use of carnitine therapy in selected cases of male factor infertility: a double-blind crossover trial. Fertil Steril. 2003;79(2):292–300.
14. Lenzi A, Picardo M, Gandini L, Dondero F. Lipids of the sperm plasma membrane: from polyunsaturated fatty acids considered as markers of sperm function to possible scavenger therapy. Hum Reprod Update. 1996;2(3):246–56.
15. Lenzi A, Sgro P, Salacone P, Paoli D, Gilio B, Lombardo F, et al. A placebo-controlled double-blind randomized trial of the use of combined l-carnitine and l-acetyl-carnitine treatment in men with asthenozoospermia. Fertil Steril. 2004;81(6):1578–84. doi:10.1016/j.fertnstert.2003.10.034.

16. Lombardo F, Sansone A, Romanelli F, Paoli D, Gandini L, Lenzi A. The role of antioxidant therapy in the treatment of male infertility: an overview. Asian J Androl. 2011;13(5):690–7. doi:10.1038/aja.2010.183.
17. Mongioi L, Calogero AE, Vicari E, Condorelli RA, Russo GI, Privitera S, et al. The role of carnitine in male infertility. Andrology. 2016; doi:10.1111/andr.12191.
18. Moradi M, Moradi A, Alemi M, Ahmadnia H, Abdi H, Ahmadi A, et al. Safety and efficacy of clomiphene citrate and L-carnitine in idiopathic male infertility: a comparative study. Urol J. 2010;7(3):188–93.
19. Mutomba MC, Yuan H, Konyavko M, Adachi S, Yokoyama CB, Esser V, et al. Regulation of the activity of caspases by L-carnitine and palmitoylcarnitine. FEBS Lett. 2000;478(1–2):19–25.
20. Pawar RS, Grundel E. Overview of regulation of dietary supplements in the USA and issues of adulteration with phenethylamines (PEAs). Drug Test Anal. 2016; doi:10.1002/dta.1980.
21. Sigman M, Glass S, Campagnone J, Pryor JL. Carnitine for the treatment of idiopathic asthenospermia: a randomized, double-blind, placebo-controlled trial. Fertil Steril. 2006;85(5):1409–14. doi:10.1016/j.fertnstert.2005.10.055.
22. Vicari E, Calogero AE. Effects of treatment with carnitines in infertile patients with prostato-vesiculo-epididymitis. Hum Reprod. 2001;16(11):2338–42.
23. Vicari E, La Vignera S, Calogero AE. Antioxidant treatment with carnitines is effective in infertile patients with prostatovesiculoepididymitis and elevated seminal leukocyte concentrations after treatment with nonsteroidal anti-inflammatory compounds. Fertil Steril. 2002; 78(6):1203–8.

Coenzyme Q10 in Male Infertility

4

Coenzyme Q10

Giancarlo Balercia, Antonio Mancini, Giacomo Tirabassi, and Alfredo Pontecorvi

4.1 Introduction

An excess of reactive oxygen species (ROS) and other oxidant radicals has been associated with male infertility [1–8]. The total oxyradical scavenging capacity (TOSC) is a recently developed assay measuring the overall capability of biological fluids or cellular antioxidants to neutralize the toxicity of various oxyradicals [9, 10]. The TOSC assay can discriminate between different forms of ROS, allowing to identify the role of specific antioxidants, or their pathway of formation in the onset of toxicological or pathological processes. The previous application of TOSC assay in andrology leads us to show a reduced antioxidant efficiency in seminal fluid of infertile men with a significant correlation between the scavenging capacity toward hydroxyl radicals and parameters of sperm cell motility [11].

Despite oxidative stress being well recognized as a cause of male infertility, the use of antioxidants as a treatment is still debated, and it is considered as a "supplementation" therapy, rather than an etiological or physiopathological therapy, since no clear correlation has been investigated between a real deficiency of a specific antioxidant and the effect of oral supplementation. Various models have been introduced to explore the protective role of different antioxidants in vitro, and some differences can be discovered regarding the protective effects exerted by specific enzymatic or non-enzymatic molecules [12]. We focus our attention on a natural antioxidant, coenzyme Q10 (CoQ10), the efficacy of which has been supported by clinical trials.

G. Balercia, MD (✉) • G. Tirabassi
Andrology Unit, Division of Endocrinology, Department of Clinical and Molecular Sciences, Via Conca 71, Umberto I Hospital, Polytechnic University of Marche, 60126 Ancona, Italy
e-mail: g.balercia@univpm.it

A. Mancini • A. Pontecorvi
Endocrinology, Catholic University of the Sacred Heart, Rome, Italy

© Springer International Publishing Switzerland 2017   43
G. Balercia et al. (eds.), *Antioxidants in Andrology*, Trends in Andrology and Sexual Medicine, DOI 10.1007/978-3-319-41749-3_4

4.2   Coenzyme Q10: Physiopathological Basis

Among natural antioxidant, a special role is covered by coenzyme Q10, also called ubiquinone for its wide distribution in different plants, animals and tissues. Coenzyme Q10, a crucial component of the mitochondrial oxidative phosphorylation process because of its role of redox, links between flavoproteins and cytochromes in the inner mitochondrial membrane; it has also many other functions, first of all the antioxidant activity, and new roles in different cellular functions were recently highlighted: this molecule can participate in redox reactions but also not in mitochondrial cellular reactions, as in lysosomes, in Golgi apparatus and in plasma membranes [13], also contributing to membrane fluidity. Moreover coenzyme Q10 can participate in many aspects of the redox control of the cellular signalling origin and transmission; in fact the autoxidation of semiquinone, formed in various membranes during electron transport, can be a primary source for H2O2 generation, which activates some transcription factors, such as NF-kB, to induce gene expression [14]. It is also possible that ROS generation could suppress other genes. There are also some indications regarding the involvement of CoQ10 in cellular proliferation at least two aspects of the stimulation of cellular proliferation concerning CoQ10 [15, 16]. Cellular growth stimulation could be based on the activation of an oxidase in the plasma membrane, which should need CoQ10 to transfer electrons through the membrane, in which is also present [17]. On the other hand, the exposition of cells to serum can induce the apoptosis, while coenzyme Q10 allows a normal cellular division. Further studies are necessary to better understand these issues.

Clinically the significance of antioxidant action of ubiquinone has been clarified by many studies concerning lipoproteins, both in vitro and in vivo. In fact LDL are molecules particularly susceptible to the oxidative damage with cytotoxic product generation, associated with vascular contractile response alterations and atherosclerosis [18]. It has been demonstrated that reduced CoQ10 present in LDL is oxidized before vitamin E and the appearance of fatty acids hydroperoxides occurs only after the oxidation of ubiquinol [19]. Moreover treatment per os with CoQ10 in normal subjects induces an increase of ubiquinol in plasma and lipoproteins and an augmented resistance to LDL peroxidation [20]. Based on the above-mentioned biochemical features, different trials have highlighted the potential therapeutic usefulness of CoQ10 in the treatment of various diseases (cardiovascular, neurologic, muscular, immunologic, diabetic endotheliopathy).

There is a relationship between low concentrations of CoQ10 and coronary pathologies, even if this correlation is not so strong to be considered a casual relation [21]. The ubiquinol/ubiquinone ratio is considered an oxidative stress marker in coronary pathologies, and the LDL/CoQ10 ratio is an index of coronary risk [22].

The role of coenzyme Q10 in influencing total antioxidant capacity (TAC) in blood plasma is supported by the significant correlation reported between these two parameters in clinical models, such as hypogonadism and hypoadrenalism [23, 24]. In these studies TAC was measured as latency phase in the formation of radicals using the system H2O2-metmyoglobin/ABTS system. On the other hand, CoQ10 levels are profoundly affected by systemic endocrine milieu, with a pivotal role for thyroid hormones [25]. Even though a clear correlation between systemic and seminal oxidative stress has been supposed but not clearly demonstrated, a possible effect of systemic thyroid hormones on semen has been also hypothesized, since seminal TAC inversely correlated with free T3 in infertile patients [26]. Finally, some therapies proposed for male infertility, such as antioestrogens, can exert their effects influencing seminal TAC [27].

Therefore, both the bioenergetic and the antioxidant roles of CoQ10 suggested a possible involvement in male fertility: it is known that a large amount of mitochondria are present in spermatozoa, in which motility requires a high energy expenditure [28]; moreover, as shown in the previous paragraph, the protection of membrane from oxidative stress could play a role in preserving sperm integrity; finally, the biosynthetic machinery for CoQ10 is present at remarkably high levels in rat testis [29].

Original studies on CoQ10 administration in unselected population of infertile patients showed an amelioration of the results in membrane integrity tests (swelling test) [30] and an improvement in seminal parameters in men with sperm pathology [31]; however, these studies did not report the endogenous CoQ10 levels in such patients.

The first analytical data on CoQ10 levels in seminal fluid were produced by our group [32], in a sample including 60 subjects (21 patients with normozoospermia, 15 patients with azoospermia or oligozoospermia, 2 patients with germ-free genital tract inflammation and 22 subjects with varicocele, 7 of whom presented oligoazoospermia). We showed that CoQ10 was assayable in total seminal fluid and in seminal plasma; its levels showed a good correlation with sperm count ($R = 0.504$, $p < 0.0005$) and motility ($R = 0.261$, $p < 0.05$), except in the population of varicocele patients, in whom the correlation with sperm count was maintained ($R = 0.666$, $p < 0.0005$) but that with sperm motility was completely lacking ($R = 0.008$, NS). Moreover, in the varicocele patients, a significantly higher proportion of total CoQ10 was present in seminal plasma when compared with normal subjects or other infertile patients without varicocele (the ratio plasma/seminal fluid Q10 was 69 ± 7.1 % vs. $41. 2 \pm. 5.6$ %, $p < 0.01$, respectively).

These data were also confirmed in larger series of patients [12, 33, 34].

Since CoQ10 in seminal plasma did not correlate with LDH levels, we concluded that the amounts of CoQ10 in plasma were not due to spermatozoa damage and to a consequent release of ubiquinone from the cells. We hypothesized that seminal plasma CoQ10 levels reflect an interchange between cellular and extracellular compartments, with a pathophysiological meaning similar to serum ubiquinone values [35, 36]; a relative deficiency or utilization of CoQ in sperm cell was therefore supposed to be present in varicocele condition [37]. We also hypothesized that the significantly higher percent of CoQ10 in plasma found in VAR patients could reflect an altered compartment distribution: the intracellular, bioenergetic use of CoQ10 could be defective in these patients, and its shift toward the plasma compartment could be considered of relevance regarding a possible antioxidant role in that environment.

Finally, we studied VAR patients, after surgical repair; only a partial reversion was observed, since the ratio plasma-to-total CoQ10 decreased, but the correlation between total CoQ10 and motility was not restored; on the contrary the peculiar correlation between cellular CoQ10 and motility was no more detectable in postoperative VAR patients [38]. Vitamin E has also been demonstrated to be positively affected by surgical VAR repair [39].

In order to explore physiological hormone control of seminal CoQ10, since FSH seemed to be involved in regulation of total antioxidant capacity of seminal plasma [40], another trial was conducted in 13 oligoasthenozoospermic subjects, studied before and after 3 months of rh-FSH (225 UI/week) [41]. Following FSH treatment, CoQ10 showed an increase, although not significant, in seminal plasma levels (0.035 ± 0.010 µg/ml vs 0.028 ± 0.005).

A recent study performed in 59 patients with idiopathic infertility failed to show a correlation between seminal plasm CoQ10 and sperm concentration or motility [42], while a correlation was present with sperm morphology; moreover the authors reported no differences between infertile patients and fertile controls. In this study however, a different method of assay was employed, an enzyme-linked immunosorbent assay (ELISA), and this could explain the different results. On the other hand, other studies proposed CoQ10, both in blood plasma and seminal fluid, together with α-tocopherol as metabolic biomarkers in both diagnosis and treatment of male infertility [43].

All these referred studies consider total CoQ10 levels, irrespective of its redox status. The first report on the assay of reduced and oxidized forms of ubiquinone was performed in our laboratory [44]. We showed a significant correlation between the reduced form (ubiquinol) and sperm count in seminal plasma, an inverse correlation between ubiquinol and hydroperoxide levels both in seminal plasma and seminal fluid, a strong correlation – using multiple regression analysis – between sperm count, motility and ubiquinol-10 content in seminal fluid, and, finally, an inverse correlation between ubiquinol/ubiquinone ratio and the percentage of abnormal forms. These results indicate an important role of ubiquinol-10 in inhibiting hydroperoxide formation. We also found a lower ubiquinol/ubiquinone ratio in sperm cells from idiopathic asthenozoospermic (IDA) patients and in seminal plasma from IDA and varicocele-associated asthenozoospermic (VARA) patients compared to controls [45]. The important conclusion was that the QH_2/Q_{OX} ratio may be an index of oxidative stress and its reduction a risk factor for semen quality. Sperm cells characterized by low motility and abnormal morphology, equipped with low CoQ10 content, could be less capable in counteracting oxidative stress, which could lead to a reduced QH_2/Q_{OX} ratio.

4.3   Coenzyme Q10: Clinical Trials

Concerning the therapeutic role of CoQ10, it should be mentioned that CoQ10 was first introduced as an ethical drug for heart failure patients, but its use has grown since its recognition as a food supplement aimed at improving cellular bioenergetics, counteracting oxidative stress and slowing down some age-related pathologies. Numerous clinical studies have shown its efficacy as an adjunctive therapy in cardiovascular and neurodegenerative diseases and in mitochondrial myopathies [46].

The above-mentioned studies constitute a rationale which eventually led us to treat infertile subjects with exogenous CoQ10.

Lewin and Lavon [47] originally reported the effect of CoQ10 on sperm motility in vitro: a significant increase in motility was observed in sperm obtained from asthenozoospermic men, incubated with exogenous CoQ10, while no significant variation was reported in the motility of sperm cells from normal subjects. The same study also reports the effect of exogenous CoQ10 in vivo, in a group of patients with low fertilization rates, after in vitro fertilization with intracytoplasmatic sperm injection for male factor infertility: no significant changes were reported in most sperm parameters, but a significant improvement was noticed in fertilization rates after a treatment with 60 mg/day for a mean of 103 days.

CoQ10 is one of the compounds contributing to the total antioxidant buffer capacity of semen, and its decrease could lead to an impairment of the system in counteracting oxidative stress [48]; exogenous administration of CoQ10 could increase its content in semen and improve sperm cell function.

In order to investigate a potential therapeutic role, we administered CoQ10 to a group of 22 idiopathic asthenozoospermic infertile patients [49], classified according to WHO 1999 criteria [50] as having < 50 % forward motile forms at two distinct sperm analyses and normal sperm morphology > 30 %.

Patients were given CoQ10 (Pharma Nord, Denmark), 200 mg/day divided into two doses, for 6 months. Semen analysis, including computer-assisted sperm analysis (CASA), and motility, CoQ10 and phosphatidylcholine assays were performed at baseline and after 6 months of therapy. A semen analysis was further performed after 6 months from interruption of therapy (wash-out). CoQ10 levels were assayed in sperm cells and seminal plasma using a Beckman Gold HPLC System (Beckman Instruments, San Ramon, CA, USA) equipped with an electrochemical detector (EC, ESA 5100, Bedford, MA, USA) [45]. PC was essentially determined according to Frei et al. [51].

An increase of CoQ10 was found in seminal plasma after treatment, the mean value rising significantly from 42.0 ± 5.1 at baseline to 127.1 ± 1.9 ng/ml after 6 months of exogenous CoQ10 administration ($p < 0.005$). A significant increase of CoQ10 content was also detected in sperm cells (from 3.1 ± 0.4 to 6.5 ± 0.3 ng/10^6 cells; $p < 0.05$). Similarly, PC levels increased significantly both in seminal plasma and sperm cells after treatment (from 1.49 ± 0.50 to 5.84 ± 1.15 µM, $p < 0.05$; and from 6.83 ± 0.98 to 9.67 ± 1.23 nmoles/10^6 cells, $p < 0.05$, respectively).

Regarding semen, a significant difference was found in forward (class a+b) motility of sperm cells after six months of CoQ10 dietary implementation (from 9.13 ± 2.50 to 16.34 ± 3.43 %, $p < 0.05$). The improvement of motility was also confirmed by means of computer-assisted determination of kinetic parameters. A significant increase of VCL (from 26.31 ± 1.50 to 46.43 ± 2.28 µm/s, $p < 0.05$) and VSL (from 15.20 ± 1.30 to 20.40 ± 2.17 µm/s, $p < 0.05$) was found after treatment. No significant differences were found in sperm cell concentration and morphology.

Although a direct correlation was not found (data not shown), a positive dependence (using Cramer's index of association) was evident among the relative variations, baseline and after treatment, of seminal plasma or intracellular CoQ10 content and of CASA (VCL and VSL) kinetic parameters (Cramer's $V = 0.4637$; 0.3818; 0.3467; 0.5148, respectively) [49].

A significant reduction in sperm forward motility was reported after 6 months of wash-out (from 16.34 ±3.43 to 9.50 ±2.28 %, $p < 0.001$), while no significant differences were found in sperm cell concentration and morphology.

In order to find out whether different responses were age related, the relative variations (before and after treatment) of CoQ10 and PC content in seminal plasma and sperm cells, as well as forward motility, were analysed, but no correlation was found (data not shown).

Wives of three out of 22 patients (13.6 %) achieved spontaneous pregnancy within 3 months from the discontinuation of therapy (2.4 % pregnancy rate per cycle).

This study indicates a significant improvement of kinetic features of sperm cells after 6 months of administration of CoQ10, both on the basis of manual and computer-assisted evaluations. Moreover, these results constitute the first demonstration that exogenous administration of CoQ10 increases its levels in seminal plasma and in spermatozoa.

The increment was important, especially in seminal plasma where post-treatment levels were three times higher than basal ones. Similar increases of CoQ10 concentration (two–three times higher than baseline value) are commonly found in blood plasma after chronic administration of the quinone [52]. As CoQ10 is a highly lipophilic molecule, we could reasonably hypothesize its diffusion through the phospholipid bilayer of cellular membranes, but we presently do not know whether transport from blood plasma to testicular and accessory male genital glands is passive or involves an active mechanism.

Statistical analysis did not reveal any significant functional relationship among the therapy-induced variations of CoQ10 and kinetic parameters of spermatozoa, probably due to the low number of samples. Nevertheless, the good degree of association among these variables, according to Cramer's V index of association, supports the hypothesis of a pathogenetic role of CoQ10 in asthenozoospermia, according to previously reported data [45, 33]. Improvement of the spontaneous pregnancy rate also suggests that this therapeutic approach is beneficial.

These results were confirmed by a double-blind, placebo-controlled clinical trial, also from our group [53]. The selected patients underwent a double-blind therapy with CoQ10 (Q-absorb soft gels, Jarrow Formulas, LA, USA), containing 100 mg of CoQ10, lecithin and medium-chain glycerides. Placebo had the same composition but the soft gels did not contain any CoQ10. All patients were given a total of two soft capsules in two separate daily administrations, with meals. The CoQ10 dose was similar to that used in our previous open trial on male infertility.

The study design was 1-month run-in, 6 months of therapy (30 patients) or placebo (30 patients) and further 3 months of follow-up (controls at months T-1, T0, T+3, T+6, T+9).

CoQ10 levels increased in seminal plasma after treatment, the mean value rising significantly from 61.29 ± 20.24 at baseline to 99.39 ± 31.51 ng/ml after 6 months of exogenous CoQ10 administration ($p < 0.0001$). A significant increase of CoQ10 content was also detected in sperm cells (from 2.44 ± 0.97 to 4.57 ± 2.46 ng/10^6 cells, $p < 0.0001$). Similarly, QH_2 levels increased significantly both in seminal plasma and sperm cells after treatment (from 31.54 ± 10.05 to 51.93 ± 16.44 ng/ml, $p < 0.0001$; and from 0.95 ± 0.46 to 1.84 ± 1.03 ng/10^6 cells, $p < 0.0001$, respectively). No statistically significant modifications were found in the placebo group.

A significant improvement of sperm cell total motility (from 33.14 ± 7.12 to 39.41 ± 6.80 %, $p < 0.0001$) and forward motility (from 10.43 ± 3.52 to 15.11 ± 7.34 %, $p = 0.0003$) was observed in the treated group after 6 months (T+6) of CoQ10 administration. The improvement of sperm cell kinetic parameters was also confirmed after computer-assisted analysis, with an increase both in VCL (from 27.99 ± 5.32 to 33.18 ± 4.22 µm/s, $p < 0.0001$) and VSL (from 10.76 ± 2.63 to 13.13 ± 2.86 µm/s, $p < 0.0001$) after treatment. No statistically significant modifications in kinetic parameters were found in placebo group.

A significant inverse correlation between baseline (T0) and T+6 relative variations of seminal plasma or intracellular CoQ10 or QH_2 content and kinetic parameters was also found in treated group. In fact patients with lower baseline value of motility and levels of CoQ10 had a statistically significant higher probability to be responders to the treatment.

After wash-out (T+9), sperm cell kinetic features (total and forward motility, VSL) resulted significantly reduced in treatment groups when compared with month T+6.

Nine spontaneous pregnancies were achieved during the observation period. After opening the randomization list, it was found that six of the patients who had impregnated their female partner had undergone CoQ10 therapy (three of them after 4 months, one after 5 months and one after 6 months of treatment). Three out of the nine pregnancies occurred in partners of patients undergoing placebo treatment, respectively, one after 2 months of therapy and the other two after 3 months of wash-out.

Recently, we reported preliminary data on effectiveness of CoQ10 treatment in improving sperm parameters in men with varicocele [54] in an open uncontrolled pilot study, performed in 38 patients. In this case, together with sperm improvement, we found a significant increase in seminal plasma TAC. Finally another retrospective study, evaluating the results in 62 infertile patients with astheno-teratozoospermia and sperm concentration greater than 13×10^6/ml, treated with 200 mg of ubiquinol, the reduced form of CoQ10, showed a significant increase in morphology and motility (fast+slow progressive cells); the authors concluded that the discrepancies reported in literature are linked to the inclusion of patients with severely diminished sperm densities, weakening the evidences in favour of CoQ10 beneficial effects [55].

The above reported controlled study [53] was inserted, in a recent meta-analysis on coenzyme Q10 and male infertility [56], together with only other two studies [57, 58], as randomized controlled studies that met inclusion criteria, excluding risk of bias as suggested by Cochrane Collaboration. The conclusion of this analysis is cautious, due to the heterogeneity of the trials: asthenozoospermia in our study and oligoasthenozoospermia in the other two studies; difference in the mean age of patients, which could be relevant considering the higher oxidation rate in advanced age; and finally different schedules of treatment were used: 100 mg twice daily in our study for 9 months, 300 mg once daily for 26 weeks [57] and 200 mg once daily for 12 weeks [58]. Despite these differences, the pooled analysis showed a significant increase in CoQ10 seminal concentrations in men who received the treatment, with higher sperm concentrations and sperm motility. Safarinejad also showed a decrease in FSH and LH and an increase in inhibin B levels, suggesting a better intratesticular sperm maturation.

The cited meta-analysis had an interest, as primary outcome, on birth and clinical pregnancy rate, which were not the primary aim of the three trials. Therefore, the conclusion is that CoQ10 induces a global improvement in sperm parameters, but additional studies are needed to give evidence to therapeutical advantage. However, other than our results above reported, also the other two studies reported in the discussion the results on pregnancy outcome. The general conclusion also can be generalized for the reviews on antioxidant employment in the therapy of male infertility [59–63].

4.4 Association of Coenzyme Q10 and Other Antioxidants

A recent observational study has been performed in a group of 20 patients affected by idiopathic asthenozoospermia, with the administration of dietary supplements including CoQ10 (200 mg) and aspartic acid (D-Asp) for a period of 3 months. D-Asp had been previously shown to increase concentration and motility [64]; in this regard, a protective effect of this molecule against OS was suggested [65]. The endpoint of the study was the evaluation not only of sperm parameters of standard semen analysis but also of DNA integrity and indexes of OS [66].

A significant increase of the administered substances, i.e. CoQ10 and D-Asp, in sperm cells and seminal fluid, respectively, was evident. Conversely, CoQ10 seminal plasma levels did not increase significantly in this experimental setting. A significant improvement of sperm kinetic parameters was observed. On the contrary, sperm count and atypical sperm cells were not affected by oral supplementation.

NO and peroxynitrite levels decreased, whereas SOD activity increased significantly after treatment. Furthermore, the percentage of damaged DNA, quantified by the index tail intensity, decreased significantly after CoQ10 and D-Asp administration.

Correlation analysis revealed a negative relationship between the increase of CoQ10 and the decrease of NO and DNA damage and a positive one between the increase of CoQ10 and the rise of SOD activity. On the contrary, no significant correlation was found between the increment of D-Asp and the changes of any of the considered markers.

Increase of SOD activity and decrease of NO levels were negatively (r, -0.456; p 0.044) and positively (r, 0.458; p 0.042) correlated with the decrease of DNA damage index, respectively, whereas no significant correlation was found between Δ-peroxynitrite and Δ-tail intensity (r, -0.266; $p > 0.05$).

The results are summarized in Tables 4.1 and 4.2.

The results of the present study seem to indicate that the protective role against DNA damage can be attributable to CoQ10 rather than D-Asp, in partial agreement with the literature [67, 68].

Table 4.1 Sperm parameters, coenzyme Q10 (CoQ10) and aspartic acid (D-Asp) levels and oxidative stress and DNA damage markers in sperm before and after treatment

	Before	After	Variation	P
Seminal CoQ$_{10}$ (µg/ml)	0.019 (0.016–0.028)	0.017 (0.007–0.068)	0.005 (−0.014–0.047)	NS
Sperm cells CoQ$_{10}$ (ng/10^6 sperm cells)	2.32 ± 1.06	7.44 ± 2.40	5.12 ± 2.38	<0.001
Seminal plasma D-Asp (µg/ml)	2.29 (1.13–3.95)	3.19 (1.93–4.87)	0.25 (−0.28–1.95)	0.022
Sperm concentration (×10^6 spermatozoa/ml)	28.5 (25.2–39.7)	40 (25.7–66.2)	3 (−6–28.2)	NS
Progressive sperm motility (%)	18 ± 8.18	24.6 ± 5.60	6.5 ± 4.29	<0.001
Total sperm motility (%)	29.8 ± 9.31	38.2 ± 4.22	8.3 ± 6.8	<0.001
Atypical sperm cells (%)	19.6 ± 7.15	16.8 ± 7.37	−2.8 ± 10.5	NS
Sperm SOD activity (units/µl)	0.008 (0.004–0.018)	0.42 (0.34–0.57)	0.41 (0.33–0.56)	<0.001
Sperm NO (µmol NO/mg protein)	121 (118.8–124.6)	57.7 (47.4–96.3)	−63.6 (−74.4 to −22.3)	<0.001
Sperm peroxynitrite (fluorescence arbitrary numbers/10^{6}cells/ml)	337.5 (275–350)	275 (250–300)	−50 (−75 to −25)	<0.001
Sperm tail intensity (%)	31 (26.2–37.7)	14 (10.5–18.5)	−16 (−21.7 to −7)	<0.001

Data are expressed as median and interquartile range or as mean and standard deviation

Abbreviations: NS not significant, *SOD* superoxide dismutase, *NO* nitric oxide

Table 4.2 Correlation analysis between significant variations of sperm coenzyme Q10 (CoQ10) and aspartic acid (D-Asp) and the significant variations of sperm oxidative stress and markers of DNA damage

	Sperm cells Δ-CoQ$_{10}$ (ng/10^6 sperm cells)	Seminal plasma Δ-D-Asp (μg/ml)
Δ-sperm SOD activity (units/μl)	r, 0.679; $p < 0.001$	NS
Δ-sperm NO (μmol NO/mg protein)	r, -0.755; $p < 0.001$	NS
Δ-sperm peroxynitrite (fluorescence arbitrary numbers/10^6 cells/ml)	NS	NS
Δ-sperm tail intensity (%)	r, -0.496; p, 0.026	NS

In the table the Pearson or Spearman correlation coefficient (r), together with the significance of the correlation (p), is reported only for significant correlations
Abbreviations: Δ-variation, *CoQ10* coenzyme Q10, *SOD* superoxide dismutase, *NO* nitric oxide, *NS* not significant

Recently [69] an improvement of DNA integrity, analysed by sperm chromatin dispersion, in patients with grade I varicocele has been observed after the administration of multivitamins (including 1500 mg L-carnitine, 60 mg vitamin C, 10 mg vitamin E, 200 mcg vitamin B9, 1 mcg vitamin B12, 10 mg zinc and 50 mcg selenium, but only 20 mg of CoQ10).

The above cited study of Gvozdjakova evaluated the effect of a mixed medication, containing 440 mg L-carnitine fumarate + 30 mg ubiquinol + 75 IU vitamin E + 12 mg vitamin C for 6 months of treatment in 40 infertile men; they observed an increase in sperm density of 39.8 % at 3 months and 78 % at 6 months of treatment; at 3 months, the sperm pathology decreased by 25.8 %. Interestingly, they showed an effect on both serum and seminal antioxidants (CoQ10, α-tocopherol) and on indexes of oxidative stress (thiobarbituric acid reactive substances). The study was not placebo controlled, however, underlining the parallelism between systemic and seminal oxidative status. Pregnancy rate obtained was 45 % (in 3 out of 18 obtained by in vitro fertilization).

Despite the combination of different antioxidants can be effective, due to a synergistic effect, it remains difficult to establish the contribution of specific molecules.

The same considerations can be made on another study performed in 169 infertile men with oligoasthenozoospermia, treated with 80 mg/day vitamin C, 40 mg/day vitamin E and 120 mg/day CoQ10 for 6 months [70]. Again significant improvement in sperm concentration and motility was reported; the treatment resulted in 28.4 % pregnancies, of which 9.5 % were spontaneous.

Conclusion

Endogenous CoQ10 is significantly related to sperm count and motility, as one could expect considering its important cellular compartmentalization; furthermore it appears to be one of the most important antioxidants in seminal plasma. Its presence in this compartment does not depend on sperm lysis, as it does not correlate with LDH [32]; moreover, its distribution between intra- and extracellular compartments seems to be an active process, which is profoundly disturbed in VAR patients [33]. CoQ10 levels in seminal plasma do correlate with sperm motility. It can be hypothesized that, in certain circumstances, the increased oxidative stress in sperm cells can somehow overconsume CoQ10 to the detriment of its bioenergetic role.

Improved sperm motility upon exogenous CoQ10 administration could be explained on the basis of the well-known involvement of CoQ10 in mitochondrial bioenergetics and of its widely recognized antioxidant properties. Regarding the first point, it is well known that mitochondrial concentration of CoQ10 in mammals is close to its K_M, as far as NADH oxidation is concerned, therefore is not kinetically saturated [71]. In these conditions, one might reasonably hypothesize that a small increase in mitochondrial CoQ10 leads to a relevant rise in respiratory velocity. The resulting improvement of oxidative phosphorylation might well affect sperm cells. Since low PC levels in semen were found to be related to a reduction of the phospholipid pool and to low antioxidant capacity [72], the increased PC content in semen after treatment might reasonably involve the restoration of scavenger equilibrium. Another possible reason for this finding is that increased levels of CoQ10 also need an appropriate, highly concentration of a lipid carrier.

Thus, the administration of CoQ10 may play a positive role in the treatment of asthenozoospermia, probably related not only to its function in mitochondrial respiratory chain but also to its antioxidant properties. The increased concentration of CoQ10 in seminal plasma and sperm cells, the improvement of semen kinetic features after treatment and the evidence of a direct correlation between CoQ10 concentrations and sperm motility strongly support a cause/effect relationship. Finally it seems to exert a protective role against oxidative damage of sperm DNA.

It remains therefore, together with carnitine, the other natural antioxidant with a demonstrated clinical usefulness [73–80], a therapy with strong physiopathological basis and not empirical basis. In this sense, the recent systematic review by Cochrane [81] underlines that the effect of oral supplementation with different antioxidants for male partners of couples undergoing assisted reproductive techniques does not induce an improvement in pregnancy rate and this objective needs to be further investigated. The role of coenzyme Q10 in oocyte maturation, mitochondrial function and female fertility is also under evaluation [82].

A deeper insight into these molecular mechanisms could lead to a greater knowledge of the so-called unexplained infertility.

References

1. Alvarez JG, Storey B. Spontaneous lipid peroxidation in rabbit epididymal spermatozoa: its effect on sperm motility. Biol Reprod. 1982;27:1102–8.
2. Aitken RJ, Clarkson JS. Cellular basis of defective sperm function and its association with the genesis of reactive oxygen species by human spermatozoa. J Reprod Fertil. 1987;81:459–69.

3. Aitken RJ, Clarkson JS, Fishel S. Generation of reactive oxygen species, lipid peroxidation and human sperm function. Biol Reprod. 1989;40:183–97.

4. Rao B, Soufir JC, Martin M, David G. Lipid peroxidation in human spermatozoa as related to midpiece abnormalities and motility. Gamete Res. 1989;24:127–34.

5. Suleiman SA, Ali ME, Zaki ZM, El-Malik EM, Nasr MA. Lipid peroxidation and human sperm motility: protective role of vitamin E. J Androl. 1996;17:530–7.

6. Aitken RJ, Krausz C. Oxidative stress, DNA damage and the Y chromosome. Reproduction. 2001;122:497–06.

7. Aitken RJ, Baker MA. Reactive oxygen species generation by human spermatozoa: a continuing enigma. Int J Androl. 2002;25:191–4.

8. Balercia G, Moretti S, Vignini A, Magagnini M, Mantero F, Boscaro M, et al. Role of nitric oxide concentration on human sperm motility. J Androl. 2004;25:245–9.

9. Winston GW, Regoli F, Dugas Jr AJ, Fong JH, Blanchard KA. A rapid chromatographic assay for determining oxyradical scavenging capacity of antioxidants and biological fluids. Free Radic Biol Med. 1998;24:480–93.

10. Regoli F, Winston GW. Quantification of total antioxidant scavenging capacity (TOSC) of antioxidants for peroxynitrite, peroxyl radicals and hydroxyl radicals. Toxicol Appl Pharmacol. 1999;156:96–105.

11. Balercia G, Mantero F, Armeni T, Principato G, Regoli F. Oxyradical scavenging capacity toward different reactive species in seminal plasma and sperm cells. A possible influence on kinetic parameters. Clin Chem Lab Med. 2003;41:13–9.

12. Mancini A, Meucci E, Bianchi A, Milardi D, De Marinis L, Littarru GP. Antioxidant systems in human seminal plasma: physiopathological meaning and new perspectives. In: Panglossi HV, editor. New perspective in antioxidant research. New York: Nova Science Pub; 2006. p. 131–47.

13. Crane FL. Biochemical functions of coenzyme Q10. J Am Coll Nutr. 2001;20(6):591–8.

14. Kaltschmidt B, Sparna T, Kaltschmidt C. Activation of NFkB by reactive oxygen intermediates in the nervous system. Antioxid Redox Signal. 1999;1:129–44.

15. Crane FL, Navas P. The diversity of coenzyme Q function. Mol Aspects Med. 1997;18:s1–6.

16. Sun IL, Sun EE, Crane FL. Comparison of growth stimulation of HeLa cells, HL-60 cells and mouse fibroblasts by coenzyme Q. Protoplasma. 1995;184:214–9.

17. Sun IL, Sun EE, Crane FL, Morrè DJ, Lindgren A, Low H. A requirement for coenzyme Q in plasma membrane electron transport. Proc Natl Acad Sci U S A. 1990;89:11126–30.

18. Thomas SR, Witting PK, Stocker R. A role for reduced coenzyme Q in atherosclerosis? Biofactors. 1999;9:207–24.

19. Stocker R, Bowry VW, Frei B. Ubiquinol-10 protects human low density lipoprotein more efficiently against lipid peroxidation than does alpha-tocopherol. Proc Natl Acad Sci U S A. 1991 Mar 1;88(5):1646–50.

20. Mohr D, Bowry VW, Stocker R. Dietary supplementation with coenzyme Q10 results in increased levels of ubiquinol-10 within circulating lipoproteins and increased resistance of human low-density lipoprotein to the initiation of lipid peroxidation. Biochim Biophys Acta. 1992 Jun 26;1126(3):247–54.

21. Yalcin A, Kilinc E, Sagcan A, Kultursay H. Coenzyme Q10 concentrations in coronary artery disease. Clin Biochem. 2004;37:706–9.

22. Mancini A, Leone E, Festa R, Grande G, Silvestrini A, De Marinis L, Pontecorvi A, Maira G, Littarru GP, Meucci E. Effects of testosterone on antioxidant systems in male secondary hypogonadism. J Androl. 2008;29(6):622–9. [E-pub 2008 Jul 17].

23. Mancini A, Leone E, Silvestrini A, Festa R, Di Donna V, De Marinis L, Pontecorvi A, Littarry GP, Meucci E. Evaluation of antioxidant systems in pituitary-adrenal axis diseases, Pituitary. Heidelberg/New York: Springer [E-pub 2009 Dec 12].

24. Hughes K, Lee BL, Feng X, Lee J, Ong CN. Coenzyme Q10 and differences in coronary heart disease risk in Asian Indians and Chinese. Free Radic Biol Med. 2002;32(2):132–8.

25. Mancini A, Festa R, Di Donna V, Leone E, Littarru GP, Silvestrini A, Meucci E, Pontecorvi A. Hormones and antioxidant systems: role of pituitary and pituitary-dependent axes. J Endocrinol Invest. 2010;33:422–33.

26. Mancini A, Festa R, Silvestrini A, Nicolotti N, Di Donna V, La Torre G, Pontecorvi A, Meucci E. Hormonal regulation of total antioxidant capacity in seminal plasma. J Androl USA. 2009;30 (5):534–540. [E-pub 2009 Feb 19].

27. Mancini A, Raimondo S, Persano M, Di Segni C, Cammarano M, Gadotti G, Silvestrini A, Pontecorvi A, Meucci E. Estrogens as antioxidant modulators in human fertility. Int J Endocrinol. (2013):607939. doi:10.1155//2013/607939. [E pub 2013 Nov 20].

28. Fawcett DW. The mammalian spermatozoon. Dev Biol. 1975;44:394–436.

29. Kalen A, Appelkvist EL, Chojnacki T, Dallner G. Nonaprenyl-4-hydroxybenzoate transferase, an enzyme involved in ubiquinone biosynthesis in endoplasmic reticulum-Golgi system of rat liver. J Biol Chem. 1990;265:1158–64.

30. Mazzilli F, Cerasaro M, Bisanti A, Rossi T, Dondero F. Seminal parameters and the swelling test in patients with sperm before and after treatment with ubiquinone (CoQ10). 2nd International symposium on reproductive medicine, Fiuggi, Rome. Acta Medica, Edizioni e Congressi, 1988, p. 71.

31. Mazzilli F, Bisanti A, Rossi T, DeSantis L, Dondero F. Seminal and biological parameters in dysspermic patients with sperm hypomotility before and after treatment with ubiquinone (CoQ10). J Endocrinol Invest 13S1. 1990;88.

32. Mancini A, De Marinis L, Oradei A, Hallgass ME, Conte G, Pozza D, Littarru GP. Coenzyme Q10 concentrations in normal and pathological human seminal fluid. J Androl. 1994;15: 591–4.

33. Mancini A, Milardi D, Conte G, Bianchi A, Balercia G, De Marinis L, Littarru GP. Coenzyme Q10: another biochemical alteration linked to infertility in varicocele patients. Metabolism. 2003;52:402–6.

34. Angelitti AG, Colacicco L, Callà C, Arizzi M, Lippa S. Coenzyme Q: potentially useful index of bioenergetic and oxidative status of spermatozoa. Clin Chem. 1995;41:217–9.

35. Mancini A, Conte G, De Marinis L, Hallgass ME, Pozza D, Oradei A, Littarru GP. Coenzyme Q10 levels in human seminal fluid: diagnostic and clinical implications. Mol Aspects Med. 1994;15:s249–55.

36. Littarru GP, Lippa S, Oradei A, Fiorini RM, Mazzanti L. Metabolic and diagnostic implications of human blood CoQ10 levels. In: Folkers K, Littarru GP, Yamagami T, editors. Biomedical and clinical aspects of coenzyme Q, vol. 6. Amsterdam: Elsevier; 1991. p. 167–78.

37. Mancini A, Conte G, Milardi D, De Marinis L, Littarru GP. Relationship between sperm cell ubiquinone and seminal parameters in subjects with and without varicocele. Andrologia. 1998;30:1–4.

38. Mancini A, Milardi D, Conte G, Festa R, De Marinis L, Littarru GP. Seminal antioxidants in humans: preoperative and postoperative evaluation of Coenzyme Q10 in varicocele patients. Horm Metab Res. 2005;37:428–32.

39. Mostafa T, Anis TH, El-Nashar A, Imam H, Othman IA. Varicocelectomy reduces reactive oxygen species levels and increases antioxidant attività of seminal plasma from infertile men with varicocele. Int J Androl. 2001;24:261–5.

40. Meucci E, Milardi D, Mordente A, Martorana GE, Giacchi E, De Marinis L, Mancini A. Total antioxidant capacity in patients with varicocele. Fertil Steril. 2003;79:1577–83.

41. A. Mancini, D. Milardi, R. Festa, G. Balercia, L. De Marinis, A. Pontecorvi, F. Principi, G.P. Littarru. Seminal CoQ10 and male infertility: effects of medical or surgical treatment on endogenous seminal plasma concentrations. Abstracts of the 4th international coenzyme Q10 association, Los Angeles, April 14–17, 2005, p. 64–5.

42. Eroglu M, Sahin S, Durukan B, Ozakpinar OB, Erdinc N, Tiurkgeldi L, Sofuoglu K, Karateke A. Blood serum and seminal plasma selenium, total antioxidant capacity and coenzyme Q10 levels in relation to semen parameters in men with idiopathic infertility. Biol Trace Elem Res. 2014;159:46–51.

43. Gvozdjakova A, Kucharska J, Dubravic J, Mojto V, Singh RB. Coenzyme Q10, α-tocopherol, and oxidative stress could be important metabolic biomarkers of male infertility. Disease Markers. 2015;ID 827941 1-6.

44. Alleva R, Scaramucci A, Mantero F, Bompadre S, Leoni L, Littarru GP. The protective role of ubiquinol-10 against formation of lipid hydroperoxides in human seminal fluid. Mol Aspects Med. 1997;18:s221–8.
45. Balercia G, Arnaldi G, Fazioli F, Serresi M, Alleva R, Mancini A, Mosca F, Lamonica GR, Mantero F, Littarru GP. Coenzyme Q10 levels in idiopathic and varicocele-associated asthenozoospermia. Andrologia. 2002;34:107–11.
46. Littarru GP, Tiano L. Clinical aspects of coenzyme Q_{10}: an update. Curr Opin Clin Nutr Metab Care. 2005;8:641–6.
47. Lewin A, Lavon H. The effect of coenzyme Q_{10} on sperm motility and function. Mol Aspects Med. 1997;18:s213–9.
48. Balercia G, Mantero F, Armeni T, Principato G, Regoli F. Oxyradical scavenging capacity toward different reactive species in seminal plasma and sperm cells. A possible influence on kinetic parameters. Clin Chem Lab Med. 2003;41:13–9.
49. Balercia G, Mosca F, Mantero F, Boscaro M, Mancini A, Ricciardo-Lamonica G, Littarru GP. Coenzyme Q(10) supplementation in infertile men with idiopathic asthenozoospermia: an open, uncontrolled pilot study. Fertil Steril. 2004;81:93–8.
50. World Health Organization (WHO). Laboratory manual for the examination of human semen and semen-cervical mucus interaction. 4th ed. Cambridge: Cambridge University Press; 1999.
51. Frei B, Yamamoto Y, Niclas D, Ames BN. Evaluation of an isoluminol chemiluminescence assay for detection of hydroperoxides in human blood plasma. Ann Biochem. 1998;175:120–30.
52. Langsjoen P, Langsjoen A, Willis R, Folkers K. Treatment of hypertrophic cardiomyopathy with coenzyme Q_{10}. Mol Aspects Med. 1997;8:145–51s.
53. Balercia G, Buldreghini E, Vignini A, Tiano L, Paggi F, Amoroso S, Ricciardo-Lamonica G, Boscaro M, Lenzi A, Littarru GP. Coenzyme Q_{10} treatment in infertile men with idiopathic asthenozoospermia: a placebo-controlled, double-blind randomized trial. Fertil Steril. 2009;91:1785–92. Bremer J. Carnitine-metabolism and functions. Physiol Rev. 1983;63:1420–80.
54. Festa R, Giacchi E, Raimondo S, Tiano L, Zuccarelli P, Silvestrini A, E.E. M, G.P. L, Mancini A. Coenzyme Q10 supplementation in infertile men with low-grade varicocele : an open, uncontrolled pilot study. Andrologia. 2013;46:805–7. doi:10.1111/and.12152. [E-pub 2013 Aug 22].
55. Cakiroglu B, Eyyupoglu SE, Gozukucuk R, Uyanik BS. Ubiquinol effect on sperm parameters in subfertile men who have astheno-teratozoospermia with normal sperm concentration. Nephro Urol Mon. 2014;6:e16870.
56. Lafuente R, Gonzalez-Comadran M, Solà I, Lopez G, Brassesco M, Carreras R, Checa MA. Coenzyme Q10 and male infertility : a meta-analysis. J Assist Reprod Genet. 2011;30:1147–56.
57. Safarinejad MR. Efficacy of coenzyme Q_{10} on semen parameters, sperm function and reproductive hormones in infertile men. J Urol. 2009;182:237–48.
58. Nadjarzadeh A, Sadeghi MR, Amirjannati N, Vafa MR, Motevalian SA, Gohari MR, et al. Coenzyme Q10 improves seminal oxidative defence but does not affect on semen parameters in idiopathic oligoasthenoteratozoospermia: a randomized double-blind, placebo controlled trial. J Endocrinol Invest. 2011;e224–8.
59. Ross C, Morriss A, Khairy M, Khalaf Y, Braude P, Coomarasamy A, El-Toukhy T. A systematic review of the effect of oral antioxidants on male infertility. Reprod Biomed Online. 2010;20:711–23. [E-pub 2010 Mar 10].
60. Lanzafame FM, La Vignera S, Vicari E, Calogero AE. Oxidative stress and medical antioxidant treatment in male infertility. Reprod Biomed Online. 2009;19:638–59.
61. Clark NA, Will M, Moravek MB, Fiseha S. A systematic review of the evidence for complementary and alternative medicine in infertility. Int J Gynaecol Obstet. 2013;122:202–6.
62. Walczak-Jedrzejowska R, Wolski JK, Slowikowska-Hilczer J. The role of oxidative stress and antioxidants in male fertility. Cent Eur J Urol. 2013;66:60–7. [E-pub 2013 Apr 26].
63. Arcaniolo D, Favilla V, Tiscione D, Pisano F, Bozzini G, Creta M, Gentile G, Menchini FF, Pavan N, Veneziano IA, Cai T, on behalf of Young Commission of Italian Andrological Society. Arch It Urol Androl. 2014;86:164–70.
64. D'Aniello G, Ronsini S, Notari T, Grieco N, Infante V, D'Angelo N, Mascia F, Di Fiore MM, Fisher G, D'Aniello A. D-aspartate, a key element for the improvement of sperm quality. Adv Sex Med. 2012;2:47–53.

65. Rathore MS, Gupta VB. Protective effect of amino acids on eye lenses against oxidative stress induced by hydrogen peroxide. As J Pharmac Clin Res. 2010;3:166–9.
66. Tirabassi G, Vignini A, Tiano L, Buldreghini E, Brugè F, Silvestri S, Orlando P, D'Aniello A, Mazzanti L, Lenzi A, Balercia G. Protective effects of coenzyme Q10 and aspartic acid on oxidative stress and DNA damage in subjects affected by idiopathic asthenozoospermia. Endocrine. 2015;(49):549–52. doi:10.3109/09537104.2014.980797. [E-pub 2014 Nov 10].
67. Talevi R, Barbato V, Fiorentino L, Braun S, Longobardi S, Gualtieri R. Protective effects of in vitro treatment with zinc, d-aspartate and coenzyme Q10 on human sperm motility, lipid peroxidation and DNA fragmentation. Reprod Biol Endocrinol. 2013;11:81. doi:10.1186/1477-7827-11-81.
68. Abad C, Amengual MJ, Gosalvez J, Coward K, Hannaoui N, Benet J, Garcia-Peirò A, Prats J. Effects of oral antioxidant treatment upon the dynamics of human sperm DNA fragmentation and subpopulations of sperm with highly degraded DNA. Andrologia. 2013;45:211–6.
69. Gual-Frau J, Abad C, Amengual MJ, Hannaoui N, Checa MA, Ribas-Maynou J, Lozano I, Nikolaou A, Benet J, Garcia-Peirò A, Prats J. Oral antioxidant treatment partly improves integrity of human sperm DNA in infertile grad I varicocele patients. Hum Fertil (Camb). 2015;18:225–9.
70. Kobori Y, Ota S, Sato R, Yagi H, Soh S, Arai G, Okada H. Antioxidant cosupplementation therapy with vitamin C, vitamin E, and coenzyme Q10 in patients with oligoasthenozoospermia. Arch It Urol Androl. 2014;86:1–4.
71. Fato R, Cavazzoni M, Castelluccio C, Parenti Castelli G, Lenaz G. Steady state kinetics of ubiquinol-cytochrome c reductase in bovine heart submitochondrial particles: diffusional effects. Biochem J. 1993;290:225–36.
72. Kelso KA, Redpath A, Noble RC, Speake BK. Lipid and antioxidant changes in spermatozoa and seminal plasma throughout the reproductive period of bulls. J Reprod Fertil. 1997;109:1–6.
73. Jeulin C, Lewin LM. Role of free L-carnitine and acetyl-L-carnitine in post-gonadal maturation of mammalian spermatozoa. Hum Reprod Update. 1996;2:87–102.
74. Balercia G, Regoli F, Armeni T, Koverech A, Mantero F, Boscaro M. Placebo-controlled double-blind randomized trial on the use of L-carnitine, L-acetylcarnitine, or combined L-carnitine and L-acetylcarnitine in men with idiopathic asthenozoospermia. Fertil Steril. 2005;84:662–71.
75. Costa M, Canale D, Filicori M, D'Iddio S, Lenzi A. L-Carnitine in idiopathic asthenozoospermia: a multicenter study. Andrologia. 1994;26:155–9.
76. Vicari E, Calogero AE. Effects of treatment with carnitines in infertile patients with prostato-vesiculo-epididymitis. Hum Reprod. 2001;16:2338–42.
77. Vicari E, La Vignera S, Calogero AE. Antioxidant treatment with carnitine is effective in infertile patients with prostato-vesiculo-epididymitis and elevated seminal leukocyte concentration after treatment with nonsteroidal anti-inflammatory compounds. Fertil Steril. 2002;78:1203–8.
78. Lenzi A, Lombardo F, Sgro P, Salacone P, Caponecchia L, Dondero F, et al. Use of carnitine therapy in selected cases of male factor infertility: a double blind cross-over trial. Fertil Steril. 2003;79:292–300.
79. Lenzi A, Sgrò P, Salacone P, Paoli D, Gilio B, Lombardo F, et al. Placebo controlled double blind randomised trial on the use of L-carnitine and L-acetyl-carnitine combined treatment in asthenozoospermia. Fertil Steril. 2004;81:1578–84.
80. Kobayashi A, Fujisawa S. Effect of L-carnitine on mitochondrial acyl-carnitine, acyl-coenzyme A and high energy phosphate in ischemic dog heart. J Mol Cell Cardiol. 1994;26:499–508.
81. Showell MG, Brown J, Yazdani A, Stankiewicz MT, Hart RJ. Antioxidants for male subfertility. Cochrane Database Syst Rev. 2011;(1):CD007411. doi: 10.1002/14651858.CD007411.pub2.
82. Ben-Meir A, Burstein E, Borrego-Alvarez A, Chong J, Wong E, Yavorska T, Naranian T, Chi M, Wang Y, Bentov Y, Alexis J, Meriano J, Sung HK, Gasser DL, Moley KH, Hekimi S, Casper RF, Jurisicova A. Coenzyme Q10 restores oocyte mitochondrial function and fertility during reproductive aging. Aging Cell. 2015;14:887–95.

Antioxidants in Male Accessory Gland Infection

5

Aldo E. Calogero, Rosita A. Condorelli, and Sandro La Vignera

5.1 Introduction

Male accessory gland infections (MAGI), also known as male accessory gland inflammation [9, 12], are characterized by infections or inflammation involving one or more of the following male genital organs or tracts [22]:

- Urethra (urethritis)
- Cowper's glands
- Prostate gland (prostatitis)
- Seminal vesicles (seminal vesiculitis)
- Epididymis (epididymitis)
- Vas deferens
- Testis (orchitis)

This condition has a negative impact on the secretory function of the male accessory glands causing alteration of the seminal fluid.

The presence of MAGI can be suspected in presence of signs of inflammation in the semen analysis (leukocytes $\geq 1 \times 10^6$/mL and/or elastase $\geq$ 230 ng/mL), low seminal volume, elevated seminal fluid pH, and low levels of alpha-glucosidase, fructose, and zinc [36].

A.E. Calogero, MD (✉) • R.A. Condorelli • S. La Vignera
Department of Clinical and Experimental Medicine, University of Catania,
Via S. Sofia 78, 95123 Catania, Italy
e-mail: acaloger@unict.it

© Springer International Publishing Switzerland 2017
G. Balercia et al. (eds.), *Antioxidants in Andrology*, Trends in Andrology
and Sexual Medicine, DOI 10.1007/978-3-319-41749-3_5

5.2   Diagnosis

The diagnosis of MAGI is made according to parameters defined by the World Health Organization (WHO). These diagnostic criteria are based on the clinical history of the patient, urogenital physical examination, and alterations of the prostate secretion and/or sperm parameters (oligo-astheno-teratozoospermia, OAT) [9, 28]. According to the WHO criteria, the diagnosis of MAGI is made when OAT is associated with:

- One factor of the group A + one factor of the group B
- One factor of the group A + one factor of the Group C
- One factor of the group B + one factor of the Group C
- Two factors of the group C

The characteristics of each group are listed in Table 5.1.

Recently, it has been proposed that elevated levels of soluble urokinase-type plasminogen activator receptor (suPAR) in seminal plasma might be useful as a marker for MAGI [3].

5.3   Clinical Presentation

The symptoms of a patient with MAGI can be investigated by collecting the clinical history. Recently, we developed a questionnaire with specific questions to investigate the presence of symptoms [23]. The questionnaire is composed

Table 5.1 Clinical and laboratory characteristics of the three groups of factors for the diagnosis of MAGI according to the WHO criteria [40]

Factor	Description
A	Clinical history of:
	Urinary tract infection
	Epididymitis
	Sexually transmitted infection
	Physical signs:
	Thickened or tender epididymis
	Tender vas deferens
	Abnormal digital rectal examination
B	Prostatic fluid:
	Abnormal prostatic secretion
	Abnormal voided urine after prostate massage
C	Seminal fluid:
	Leukocytes $\geq 1 \times 10^6$/mL
	Seminal fluid culture with significant growth of pathogenic bacteria
	Abnormal semen appearance
	Increased semen viscosity
	Increased pH
	Abnormal biochemistry of the seminal plasma

of 30 questions with four possible answers, subdivided in four symptom domains:

1. Urination: urinary frequency, nocturia, urgent need to urinate, dysuria, pain during urination, etc.
2. Ejaculation: pain/discomfort during or after ejaculation in the suprapubic and/or perineal, reduced ejaculation volume, hemospermia, chronic pelvic pain, etc.
3. Sexual sphere: reduction of the ability to achieve and/or maintain a satisfactory degree of penile rigidity and premature or delayed ejaculation
4. Quality of life: significant reduction of quality of life

Infertile patients with prostate-vesiculitis or prostate-vesiculo-epididymitis have higher questionnaire scores compared to patients with prostatitis alone. In addition, patients with prostate-vesiculo-epididymitis show high scores in domains number 2 and 3 compared to patients with prosto-vesiculitis, confirming that the greater extent of inflammation correlates with symptoms [23]. Potential complications of MAGI are [9, 12, 22, 36]:

- Obstruction of the epididymis
- Impairment of spermatogenesis
- Impairment of sperm function
- Induction of sperm autoantibodies
- Dysfunctions of the male accessory glands

These complications can result in sexual dysfunction [9, 12] and male subfertility [24, 28].

5.4 Classification

According to the extension, MAGI can be classified in uncomplicated and complicated forms. The former include prostatitis, whereas the latter comprehend prostate-vesiculitis, prostate-vesiculo-epididymitis, and epididymo-orchitis. Moreover, according to the presence/absence of microorganisms, MAGI can be divided into microbial, characterized by the presence of bacteria, fungi, and virus, and inflammatory forms, characterized by leukocytospermia and/or overproduction of reactive oxygen species (ROS).

MAGI microbial forms show the growth of more than 10^3 pathogenic bacteria or more than 10^4 nonpathogenic bacteria per ml, in culture of diluted seminal plasma. The most common microorganisms are *Enterobacteriaceae* (such as *Escherichia coli* and *Klebsiella*), *Neisseria gonorrhoeae*, and *Chlamydia trachomatis* [22]. A recent study has shown that patients with MAGI who have lower serum levels of total testosterone tend to have a more complicated form of MAGI, involving more than one site, than those with normal levels [9, 12].

According to the National Institutes of Health classification (category II), some Gram-negative bacteria (*Enterobacteriaceae* such as *Escherichia coli, Klebsiella* species, *Proteus, Serratia, Pseudomonas* species, etc.) and etiological agents of sexually transmitted diseases (*Chlamydia trachomatis, Ureaplasma urealyticus, Treponema pallidum, Neisseria gonorrhoeae*, etc.) are acknowledged as "certain pathogens" of the prostate.

Gram-positive germs (*Enterococcus* spp., *Staphylococcus aureus*, and obligate anaerobes) or coagulase-negative germs (*Staphylococcus haemolyticus, Staphylococcus epidermidis*, and mycoplasmas) are occasionally detectable in the urogenital tract and are considered by some authors to be "nonpathogenic" [27].

A viral form emerging seems to be the HPV infection [29] that, therefore, cannot rely on antibiotic treatment.

5.5   Treatment of Microbial Forms of MAGI

Antibiotics are prescribed when a urogenital infection is identified. Negative culture may occur for various reasons: low sample volume, antibiotic treatment prior to collection of the prostate secretions, and presence of undetectable microorganisms. These patients, with clinical evidence of chronic prostatitis, may also benefit from antibiotic treatment to improve the symptomatology.

The antibiotic must have a higher dissociation constant to allow its diffusion into the prostate because of the epithelial lining and pH gradient that inhibit this transition. A meta-analysis of randomized, controlled trials on the pharmacologic treatment of chronic prostatitis and chronic pelvic pain syndrome showed that α-blockers and antibiotics, as well as combinations of these drugs, appear to achieve the greatest improvement in clinical symptom scores, compared with placebo [2]. Anti-inflammatory drugs had a lower, but measurable, benefit on selected outcomes [18].

The most used antibiotics in the clinical practice are quinolones (ciprofloxacin, levofloxacin, etc.), tetracyclines, macrolides, trimethoprim, and β-lactam antibiotics (penicillin derivatives, cephalosporins, monobactams, carbapenems) [34, 39]. The addition of anti-inflammatory drugs and α-blockers (terazosin, doxazosin) improves symptoms. The α-blockers can help to decrease recurrences by diminishing urinary obstruction due to prostate enlargement or congestion secondary to inflammation.

Complicated MAGI are characterized by a chronic inflammatory response and oxidative stress-related alterations. In these cases, a better sperm response is obtained from the sequential treatment strategy: antibiotics (if needed) followed by anti-inflammatory drugs and subsequent antioxidant prescription [44, 45].

5.6   Treatment of Inflammatory Forms of MAGI

The inflammatory forms are characterized by leukocytospermia (seminal fluid leukocyte concentration $>10^6$/ml) and/or overproduction of ROS.

An increased number of leukocytes in the seminal fluid may persist even after antibiotic treatment for a microbial form in some patients with complicated MAGI, such as prostate-vesiculo-epididymitis. In addition to leukocytospermia [49], these patients have often abnormal conventional sperm parameters (concentration, motility, and morphology) [50] and other signs of inflammation. Anti-inflammatory drugs should be given when leukocytospermia and/or inflammatory sign and/or symptoms are present. The main anti-inflammatory drugs include nonsteroidal anti-inflammatory drugs (salicylates, fenamic acids, profens, Cox-2 inhibitors, arylacetics, sulfonanilides, oxicams), steroidal anti-inflammatory drugs, and fibrinolytic treatment (serratiopeptidase, bromelain, escin).

MAGI can cause infertility with multiple pathogenetic mechanisms that act at different levels to damage spermatozoa. The infectious/inflammatory process can damage spermatozoa directly or in an indirect manner by altering their microenvironment or determining a sub-obstruction of the excretory proximal and/or distal seminal tract where they transit toward the outside.

The conventional sperm parameters (concentration, motility, and morphology) are frequently altered. MAGI may also affect negatively the so-called biofunctional sperm parameters increasing the percentage of spermatozoa with fragmented DNA, with low mitochondrial membrane potential and apoptosis, and decreasing the number of viable spermatozoa [25].

Most of the studies seem to confirm that MAGI are an important risk factor for male infertility [25]. MAGI are also frequently associated with pH changes, increased seminal fluid liquefaction time, presence of macrophages, sperm aggregations, sperm agglutination, and debris [26]. The greater is the extension of MAGI, the higher is their negative impact on sperm parameters. Therefore, patients with prostate-vesiculo-epididymitis have significantly worst sperm parameters compared to patients with prostatitis alone or prostate-vesiculitis who experience only slight effects on sperm parameters [43]. In addition, we subsequently showed that patients with bilateral prostate-vesiculo-epididymitis have sperm parameters significantly worse than patients with unilateral prostate-vesiculo-epididymitis [46]. Moreover, infertile patients with hypertrophic-congestive MAGI have a better sperm quality but higher oxidative stress in semen compared to patients with fibrosclerotic MAGI. [28]. Altogether, these findings suggest that patients with MAGI and particularly those with complicated MAGI who seek fertility benefit from antioxidant prescription.

5.7 Antioxidants

Antioxidants can be used both in microbial and inflammatory forms of MAGI with different sequential treatment strategy after removal of the prooxidant factors, such as germs and/or leukocytes [44, 45].

The protective antioxidant system comprehends enzymatic factors that interact with each other to ensure an optimal protection against the oxidative stress. A deficiency of one of them may result in a decrease of total plasma antioxidant capacity [47].

The main antioxidant commercially available or currently used is discussed below, whereas other used compounds are reported in Table 5.2.

Table 5.2 Other antioxidants

Micronutrients	Selenium, zinc, copper
Amino acids	Arginine, taurine, ornithine, citrulline
Vitamins	Vitamins of group B complex, niacin (vitamin PP), pantothenic acid, folic acid
Omega-3 fatty acids	Docosanoic acid (DHA), eicosanoid acid (EPA)
Others	Magnesium, flavonoid, superoxide dismutase, *Serenoa repens*, Astaxantina, *Curcuma longa*, *Camellia sinensis*, *Urtica dioica*, *Lepidium meyenii Walp.*, muira puama (*Ptychopetalum olacoides Benth*), *Ginkgo biloba*, *Scutellaria baicalensis Georgi* and *Radix*, *Pinus massoniana*, *Cucurbita maxima*, *Aesculus hippocastanum*, *Crocus sativus*, *Epilobium* (*angustifolium* and *parviflorum*), *Citrus bergamia*, *Ortosiphon*, etc.
Other combined therapies	Vitamin E + selenium, vitamin C + vitamin E, NAC + vitamin A + vitamin E + essential fatty acids, selenium + NAC, vitamin A + vitamin E + astaxanthin

5.7.1 Glutathione

Glutathione is present both in a reduced (GSH) and in an oxidized (GSSG) state. It is a sulfur-containing tripeptide. GSH is an electron donor to glutathione peroxidase, while GSH levels are synthesized de novo or recycled by glutathione reductase, using NADPH as an electron donor. GSH displays its antioxidant activity by the reconstruction of thiol groups (−SH) in proteins and preventing cell membrane from lipid oxidation [47].

Some authors suggested that its supplementation plays a therapeutic role in some andrological diseases, particularly during inflammation. Accordingly, its supplementation in infertile men with unilateral varicocele or inflammation of the urogenital tract leads to a significant improvement of sperm parameters, such as concentration, motility, and morphology [21], as well as an improvement of the symptomatology.

Glutathione is given at the dosage of 600 mg/day intramuscularly for 2–3 months. However, the route of administration lowers its compliance.

5.7.2 Carnitine

Carnitine is the molecule with antioxidant activity that has the greatest consensus in literature. It exists as L-carnitine and L-acetylcarnitine.

L-carnitine, mainly of exogenous origin, acts as an essential cofactor for the transport of long-chain fatty acids within the mitochondrial matrix in order to facilitate the oxidative processes and to enhance cellular energy production [1, 38]. It is a high-polar, water-soluble quaternary amine. High concentrations of carnitine are present in the epididymis, suggesting its crucial role in energy metabolism and sperm maturation [30], and some studies have shown a decreased L-carnitine concentration in the seminal fluid of patients with epididymitis [6].

Since patients with prostate-vesiculo-epididymitis have the highest levels of oxidative stress, some studies have evaluated the antioxidant properties of L-carnitine administration in patients with this form of MAGI. The results of these studies have shown that the best effect is obtained administering first antibiotics, since they had initially a urogenital infection, and anti-inflammatory drugs and subsequently L-carnitine [44, 45]. Antioxidant treatment with carnitines is effective in patients with abacterial PVE and improves seminal leukocyte concentrations if these patients have been pretreated with nonsteroidal anti-inflammatory drugs [45].

Moreover, the treatment with acetyl-L-carnitine increases sperm motility and viability in asymptomatic infertile patients with ROS overproduction and ultrasonographic evidence of prostate-vesiculo-epididymitis who already received antimicrobial therapy [44]. However, although improving sperm parameters, no statistical significant variation of seminal plasma α-glycosidase concentration (a marker of epididymal function) and of sperm membrane lipid peroxidation [31] was observed. The coadministration of L-carnitine (2 g/day) and acetyl-L-carnitine (500 mg twice a day) is also effective in improving sperm quality in infertile patients [32], and it increases the total oxyradical scavenging capacity of the seminal fluid [5] and sperm parameters [14].

The best therapeutic scheme is represented by the coadministration of at least 2 g/daily of L-carnitine and at least 1 g/daily of acetyl-L-carnitine for at least 3 months.

5.7.3 N-Acetylcysteine

N-acetylcysteine is a glutathione precursor and is effective in metal chelation. It seems to prevent sperm DNA oxidative damage [47]. In an animal model, it is able to improve seminal vesicle weight, previously altered by treatment with As_2O_3 [13]. Furthermore, it significantly improves seminal fluid volume and viscosity and increases sperm motility in humans [8]. N-acetylcysteine ameliorates the carrageenan-induced prostatitis and prostate inflammation pain through miR-141 regulating Keap1/Nrf2 signaling [48].

The most common oral dosage used is 600 mg/day for at least 3 months. It is commercialized in combination with other antioxidants.

5.7.4 Coenzyme Q10

Coenzyme Q10 is present in three redox states: ubiquinone (CoQ10-oxidized), ubiquinol (CoQ10H2-reduced), and semiquinone (partially reduced, as radical). It inhibits protein and DNA oxidation and lipid peroxidation regulating the mitochondrial electron transport in the respiratory chain [20]. The reduced form has a higher antioxidant effect and concentration in the body is approximately 90 % of the total coenzyme Q10.

Coenzyme Q10 has been shown to improve sperm parameters (concentration, motility, and morphology) in men with idiopathic OAT [4, 41]. In addition, its administration improves sperm parameters and the antioxidant status in infertile men with varicocele [20]. Positive effects on sperm parameters have been obtained by higher dosages (e.g., 100–600 mg/die) [20].

Ubiquinol has a stronger antioxidant action in comparison with ubiquinone. Coenzyme Q10 levels are present in sperm thanks to an active testicular biosynthesis [35]. Ubiquinol sperm concentration strongly correlates with sperm count, motility, and morphology. In addition, coenzyme Q10 total concentration directly correlates with sperm motility [20]. Ubiquinol is administered orally at a dosage of 150–200 mg daily, for at least 4 months.

5.7.5 Vitamin A

Carotenoid is a group of fat-soluble organic compounds found mainly in yellow, red, orange, and pink vegetables. Vitamin A derives from retinoids. It seems to protect cell membrane integrity, to regulate epithelial cell proliferation, and is involved in the regulation of spermatogenesis with various effects on fetal and neonatal Sertoli, germ, and Leydig cells [33, 47]. Not many studies have evaluated the effects of vitamin A on male urogenital tract.

5.7.6 Vitamin C (Ascorbic Acid)

Vitamin C has a more powerful antioxidant action when peroxy radicals are present in the aqueous phase [17] and then in the lipid membrane [15]. In mice, at a concentration equivalent to the human therapeutic dose (10 mg/kg), it is able to reduce MDA concentration, increasing sperm count and the proportion of normal sperm population [37]. The majority of the studies reported in literature investigate the effect of vitamin C administration on sperm quality, but there is no evidence of its administration in patients with MAGI.

5.7.7 Vitamin E

Vitamin E (α-tocopherol) protects sperm cell membrane from oxidative stress-induced damage, preventing lipid peroxidation and capturing free hydroxyl radicals and superoxide [47]. A placebo-controlled double-blind study reported an improvement of sperm motility in men with OAT after vitamin E oral supplementation. The enhancement of sperm motility was associated with a decreased sperm production of MDA, a lipid peroxidation end product [42]. Finally, dietary habits seem also to play a role in semen quality, since a positive correlation has been found between vitamin E dietary intake and progressive and total motility [16]. This evidence suggests that vitamin E may have a positive effect on semen quality.

5.7.8 Myoinositol

Inositol is a precursor of second messengers and it is involved in several signal trans-duction mechanisms in the cell membrane. Inositols are involved in sperm capacitation and acrosome reaction. Myoinositol regulates seminal plasma osmolarity and volume and the expression of proteins essential for sperm chemotaxis and sperm motility.

There are no scientific evidences about the administration of myoinositol in patients with MAGI, but in both normozoospermic men and in patients with abnor-mal sperm parameters, the incubation with myoinositol results in an increased sperm motility and in a higher number of spermatozoa retrieved by swim-up. Moreover, it has been shown an improvement of sperm mitochondrial function in patients with OAT [10, 11]. A double-blind, randomized, placebo-controlled study showed that patients with idiopathic infertility, treated for 3 months with myoinosi-tol (2 g twice daily), had a significant increase of sperm concentration, total count, progressive motility, and acrosome-reacted spermatozoa [7]. The recommended daily oral dose is 4 g (plus 400 µg of folic acid), for at least 2 months.

5.7.9 Lycopene

Few studies investigated effects of lycopene on sperm parameters. Its oral adminis-tration (2 g twice a day for 3 months) improved sperm concentration and motility [19]. Various lycopene supplementation studies conducted on both humans and ani-mals have shown a decrease of lipid peroxidation and DNA damage and an improve-ment of sperm count and viability with a reduction of the oxidative stress. Further studies are required to determine the dosage and the usefulness of lycopene in this field and particularly in patients with MAGI.

5.7.10 Zinc

Zinc supplements have been suggested as a medical therapy in patients with MAGI because a zinc-containing polypeptide called prostatic antibacterial factor (PAF) may be an important prostate antimicrobial factor. Zinc is given orally at the dose of 220 mg once or twice a day for 3 to 4 months, alone or in addition to folic acid (5 mg daily). In combined therapies, it is administered at the dose of at least 10 mg a day.

References

1. Agarwal A, Virk G, Ong C, et al. Effect of oxidative stress on male reproduction. World J Mens Health. 2004;32:1–17.
2. Anothaisintawee T, Attia J, Nickel JC, et al. Management of chronic prostatitis/chronic pelvic pain syndrome: a systematic review and network meta-analysis. JAMA. 2011;305:78–86.
3. Autilio C, Morelli R, Milardi D, et al. Soluble urokinase-type plasminogen activator receptor as a putative marker of male accessory gland inflammation. Andrology. 2015;3:1054–61.

4. Balercia G, Buldreghini E, Vignini A, et al. Coenzyme Q10 treatment in infertile men with idiopathic asthenozoospermia: a placebo-controlled, double-blind randomized trial. Fertil Steril. 2009;91:1785–92.

5. Balercia G, Regoli F, Armeni T, et al. Placebo-controlled double-blind randomized trial on the use of L-carnitine, L-acetylcarnitine, or combined L-carnitine and L-acetylcarnitine in men with idiopathic asthenozoospermia. Fertil Steril. 2005;84:662–71.

6. Bornman MS, du Toit D, Otto B, et al. Seminal carnitine, epididymal function and spermatozoal motility. S Afr Med J. 1989;75:20–1.

7. Calogero AE, Gullo G, La Vignera S, et al. Myoinositol improves sperm parameters and serum reproductive hormones in patients with idiopathic infertility: a prospective double-blind randomized placebo-controlled study. Andrology. 2015;3:491–5.

8. Ciftci H, Verit A, Savas M, et al. Effects of N-acetylcysteine on semen parameters and oxidative/antioxidant status. Urology. 2009;74:73–6.

9. Condorelli RA, Calogero AE, Vicari E, et al. Male accessory gland infection: relevance of serum total testosterone levels. Int J Endocrinol. 2014;2014:915752.

10. Condorelli RA, La Vignera S, Bellanca S, et al. Myoinositol: does it improve sperm mitochondrial function and sperm motility? Urology. 2012;79:1290–5.

11. Condorelli RA, La Vignera S, Di Bari F, et al. Effects of myoinositol on sperm mitochondrial function in-vitro. Eur Rev Med Pharmacol Sci. 2011;15:129–34.

12. Condorelli RA, Vicari E, Calogero AE, et al. Male accessory gland inflammation prevalence in type 2 diabetic patients with symptoms possibly reflecting autonomic neuropathy. Asian J Androl. 2014;16:761–6.

13. da Silva RF, dos Santos BC, Villela P, et al. The coadministration of N-acetylcysteine ameliorates the effects of arsenic trioxide on the male mouse genital system. Oxid Med Cell Longev. 2016;2016:4257498.

14. De Rosa M, Boggia B, Amalfi B, et al. Correlation between seminal carnitine and functional spermatozoal characteristics in men with semen dysfunction of various origins. Drugs R D. 2005;6:1–9.

15. Doba T, Burton GW, Ingold KU. Antioxidant and co-antioxidant activity of vitamin C. The effect of vitamin C, either alone or in the presence of vitamin E or a water-soluble vitamin E analogue, upon the peroxidation of aqueous multilamellar phospholipid liposomes. Biochim Biophys Acta. 1985;835:298–303.

16. Eskenazi B, Kidd SA, Marks AR, et al. Antioxidant intake is associated with semen quality in healthy men. Hum Reprod. 2005;20:1006–12.

17. Frei B, England L, Ames BN. Ascorbate is an outstanding antioxidant in human blood plasma. Proc Natl Acad Sci U S A. 1989;86:6377–81.

18. Gill BC, Shoskes DA. Bacterial prostatitis. Curr Opin Infect Dis. 2016;29:86–91.

19. Gupta NP, Kumar R. Lycopene therapy in idiopathic male infertility – a preliminary report. Int Urol Nephrol. 2002;34:369–72.

20. Gvozdjáková A, Kucharská J, Dubravicky J, et al. Coenzyme Q10, α-tocopherol, and oxidative stress could be important metabolic biomarkers of male infertility. Dis Markers. 2015;2015:827941.

21. Irvine DS. Glutathione as a treatment for male infertility. Rev Reprod. 1996;1:6–12.

22. Krause WKH. Male accessory gland infection. Andrologia. 2008;40:113–6.

23. La Vignera S. Male accessory gland infections: anatomical extension of inflammation and severity of symptoms evaluated by an original questionnaire. Andrologia. 2012;44:739–46.

24. La Vignera S, Condorelli R, D'Agata R, et al. Semen alterations and flow-cytometry evaluation in patients with male accessory gland infections (MAGI). J Endocrinol Invest. 2012;35:219–23.

25. La Vignera S, Condorelli RA, Vicari E, et al. High frequency of sexual dysfunction in patients with male accessory gland infections. Andrologia. 2012;44:438–46.

26. La Vignera S, Condorelli RA, Vicari E, et al. Hyperviscosity of semen in patients with male accessory gland infection: direct measurement with quantitative viscosimeter. Andrologia. 2012c;44:556–9.

27. La Vignera S, Condorelli RA, Vicari E, et al. Microbiological investigation in male infertility: a practical overview. J Med Microbiol. 2014;63:1–14.

28. La Vignera S, Vicari E, Condorelli RA, et al. Hypertrophic-congestive and fibro-sclerotic ultrasound variants of male accessory gland infection have different sperm output. J Endocrinol Invest. 2011;34:330–5.
29. La Vignera S, Vicari E, Condorelli RA, et al. Prevalence of human papilloma virus infection in patients with male accessory gland infection. Reprod Biomed Online. 2015;30:385–91.
30. Lenzi A, Lombardo F, Gandini L, et al. Metabolism and action of L-carnitine: its possible role in sperm tail function. Arch Ital Urol Nefrol Androl. 1992;64:187–96.
31. Lenzi A, Lombardo F, Sgrò P, et al. Use of carnitine therapy in selected cases of male factor infertility: a double-blind crossover trial. Fertil Steril. 2003;79:292–300.
32. Lenzi A, Sgrò P, Salacone P, et al. A placebo-controlled double-blind randomized trial of the use of combined l-carnitine and l-acetyl-carnitine treatment in men with asthenozoospermia. Fertil Steril. 2004;81:1578–84.
33. Livera G, Rouiller-Fabre V, Durand P, et al. Multiple effects of retinoids on the development of Sertoli, germ, and Leydig cells of fetal and neonatal rat testis in culture. Biol Reprod. 2000;62:1303–14.
34. Magri V, Montanari E, Škerk V, et al. Fluoroquinolone-macrolide combination therapy for chronic bacterial prostatitis: retrospective analysis of pathogen eradication rates, inflammatory findings and sexual dysfunction. Asian J Androl. 2011;13:819–27.
35. Mancini A, Conte G, Milardi D, et al. Relationship between sperm cell ubiquinone and seminal parameters in subjects with and without varicocele. Andrologia. 1998;30:1–4.
36. Marconi M, Pilatz A, Wagenlehner F, et al. Impact of infection on the secretory capacity of the male accessory glands. Int Braz J Urol. 2009;35:299–308.
37. Mishra M, Acharya UR. Protective action of vitamins on the spermatogenesis in lead-treated Swiss mice. J Trace Elem Med Biol. 2004;18:173–8.
38. Ng CM, Blackman MR, Wang C, et al. The role of carnitine in the male reproductive system. Ann N Y Acad Sci. 2004;1033:177–88.
39. Perletti G, Marras E, Wagenlehner FM, et al. Antimicrobial therapy for chronic bacterial prostatitis. Cochrane Database Syst Rev. 2013;CD009071.
40. Rowe P, Comhaire F, Hargreave TB, et al. World Health Organization manual for the standardised investigation and diagnosis of the infertile couple. Cambridge: Cambridge University Press; 1993.
41. Safarinejad MR. Efficacy of coenzyme Q10 on semen parameters, sperm function and reproductive hormones in infertile men. J Urol. 2009;182:237–48.
42. Suleiman SA, Ali ME, Zaki ZM, et al. Lipid peroxidation and human sperm motility: protective role of vitamin E. J Androl. 1996;17:530–7.
43. Vicari E. Seminal leukocyte concentration and related specific radical oxygen species production in different categories of patients with male accessory gland infections. Hum Reprod. 1999;14:2025–30.
44. Vicari E, Calogero AE. Effect of treatment with carnitines in patients with prostato-vesiculo-epididymitis. Hum Reprod. 2001;16:2338–42.
45. Vicari E, La Vignera S, Calogero AE. Antioxidant treatment with carnitines is effective in infertile patients with prostato-vesiculo-epididymitis and elevated seminal leukocyte concentration after treatment with non-steroidal anti-inflammatory compounds. Fertil Steril. 2002;78:1203–8.
46. Vicari E, La Vignera S, Garrone F, et al. Terapia ormonale e non ormonale nell'infertilità maschile: indicazione e nuove prospettive. Contraccezione, Fertilità e Sessualità. 2006;33:236–42.
47. Walczak-Jedrzejowska R, Wolski JK, Slowikowska-Hilczer J. The role of oxidative stress and antioxidants in male fertility. Cent Eur J Urol. 2013;66:60–7.
48. Wang LL, Huang YH, Yan CY, et al. N-acetylcysteine ameliorates prostatitis via miR-141 regulating Keap1/Nrf2 signaling. Inflammation. 2016;39:938–47.
49. World Health Organization. WHO laboratory manual for the examination and processing of human semen. 5th ed. Geneva; World Health Organization; 2010.
50. Yanushpolsky EH, Politch JA, Hill JA, et al. Is leukocytospermia clinically relevant? Fertil Steril. 1996;66:822.

Antioxidants in Male Sexual Dysfunctions

6

Andrea Sansone, Emmanuele A. Jannini, and Francesco Romanelli

6.1 Male Sexual Dysfunctions

Andrological evaluation is aimed to assess the presence and the degree of male sexual dysfunction. This term includes some conditions that, while being separate from each other, might often coexist [25, 28]. Premature ejaculation (PE) and erectile dysfunction (ED) are the two most prevalent sexual dysfunctions; delayed ejaculation and hypoactive sexual desire, on the other hand, are at the other end of the spectrum, being less common and generally perceived as temporary disturbances. Treatment for sexual dysfunctions has been vastly investigated in the last decades, with the introduction of phosphodiesterase type 5 (PDE-5) inhibitors giving new fuel to research: to date, despite the widespread use of existing medications, the quest for new therapies hasn't ended yet.

On the other hand, priapism is a completely different male sexual dysfunction: despite being a medical and surgical emergency in most circumstances, antioxidant treatment might play a role in prevention of recurrences.

Reactive oxygen species (ROS) play a role in most biological processes, ranging from transcription factor activation to ion transport systems activity and from immune response to platelet activation [56]. Given that oxidative stress is virtually ubiquitous and undiagnosable in the routine evaluation and that administration of ROS scavengers is relatively free from side effects, antioxidant treatment has been proposed as a substitute or an addition to existing therapies for male sexual dysfunctions.

A. Sansone • F. Romanelli (✉)
Sapienza – University of Rome, Department of Experimental Medicine,
Section of Medical Pathophysiology, Food Science and Endocrinology,
Rome, Italy
e-mail: francesco.romanelli@uniroma1.it

E.A. Jannini
Tor Vergata University of Rome, Department of Systems Medicine, Rome, Italy

© Springer International Publishing Switzerland 2017
G. Balercia et al. (eds.), *Antioxidants in Andrology*, Trends in Andrology and Sexual Medicine, DOI 10.1007/978-3-319-41749-3_6

6.2   Premature Ejaculation

As premature ejaculation (PE) is a "culture-dependent symptom that is self-identified, self-reported, and self-rated" [48], consistent evidence in regard to its exact prevalence is lacking. However, reports conclude that PE is the most prevalent male sexual dysfunction [15], affecting between 8 and 30 % [24] or 22–38 % [37] of men of all ages. Different definitions of PE have been proposed by scientific societies based on time of onset, pathogenesis, and situational occurrence: however, there is an agreement in regard to the presence of brief ejaculatory latency, loss of control, and psychological distress in the patient and/or partner [38]. Biological and psychological factors are involved in the pathogenesis of PE: searching for a true "Manichean" distinction between organic and psychogenic forms of this symptom is often unhelpful [27]. Treatment is rarely sought after by the patients: PE is in fact the only partner-oriented male sexual dysfunction [36] and is therefore a symptom exclusively occurring in the couple.

6.2.1   Oxidative Stress and Premature Ejaculation

The role of oxidative stress in the pathogenesis of PE hasn't been extensively studied; this is hardly surprising, considering that the exact pathophysiology of ejaculation is far from fully understood. It has been observed that nitric oxide (NO) levels in men with PE are significantly lower than in healthy controls [44]; previous reports hinted at increased expression of antioxidant enzymes in patients compared to healthy subjects [3]. Evaluation in seminal plasma has shown lower magnesium concentrations in men with PE: hypothetically, this might result in decreased nitric oxide, in increased endothelial intracellular Ca^{2+}, and ultimately in premature emission and ejaculation [43]. It's still too early to understand whether antioxidants might be helpful in treating or even preventing PE: to the present date, scientific literature provides no definite evidence in support of or against treatment with antioxidants.

However, some of the conditions frequently associated with PE might benefit from the administration of these drugs. Prostate enlargement is common – perhaps the most common among the lower urinary tract symptoms (LUTS) – and is a frequent correlate of premature ejaculation [16]. Oxidative stress plays a pivotal role in LUTS: many drugs routinely used for their treatment act as antioxidants, including *Serenoa repens* [23], proving that at least in theory there is the chance that improving ROS-scavenging mechanisms might have a positive effect on PE.

6.3   Erectile Dysfunction

Erectile dysfunction (ED), on the other hand, is a somewhat rarer sexual dysfunction, although it's perceived as a significant health issue by those affected [51]. ED is defined as the inability to achieve or maintain erections sufficient for satisfactory sexual intercourse [42]; its prevalence is increasing with age, from 1 to 10 % in men younger than 40 and up to 70–100 % in men older than 70 years [34, 46]. Erectile dysfunction can be classified according to the clinical severity from the subclinical (but still deserving clinical attention) to more severe forms [26]. Once considered a psychogenic disease, ED has undergone extensive research which has proven its multifactorial, organic origin in a vast majority of patients [14, 50, 55]. ED is not a disease per se; more commonly, it is only a symptom of an underlying disease, whose outcomes can be far more hazardous [21]. Endocrine alterations [22, 47] can be involved in the pathogenesis of ED, although cardiovascular conditions and metabolic syndrome are more prevalent in the general population [4, 30].

6.3.1   The Role of Nitric Oxide in the Pathophysiology of Erection

Nitric oxide (NO) is considered the key molecule for erectile mechanisms: the NO/cGMP cascade is the main control system for penile erection [7], and reports in regard to its role in the pathophysiology of ED are increasing by the day. NO acts on relaxation of penile vasculature and penile smooth muscle via the cyclic guanosine monophosphate pathway. NO is produced by the enzyme NO synthase (NOS) via oxidization of L-arginine, NADPH, and oxygen, leaving L-citrulline as a by-product and using several cofactors, including tetrahydrobiopterin and calmodulin. Endothelial NOS (eNOS) and neuronal NOS (nNOS) are constitutively expressed, are bound to Ca^{2+} and calmodulin, and are the two forms mainly involved with erectile function; an inducible third isoform, defined iNOS, independent of Ca^{2+} and calmodulin and requiring new protein synthesis, is believed to be expressed in response to cellular stress – including cells from the penile vascular bed [40]. The three isoforms are synthesized as monomers and can catalyze production of NO from its substrate L-arginine only when coupled.

After its release by nNOS in nerve terminals or by eNOS in endothelial cells, NO diffuses to the smooth muscle cells of the corpora cavernosa where it raises intracellular cGMP levels by activating the soluble form of guanylate cyclase: this molecular pathway ultimately results in achievement of erection (Fig. 6.1). It is therefore clear that any condition resulting in impaired function and responsiveness of the cavernosal vascular bed – including diabetes mellitus, hypertension, and aging – might lead to reduced erectile function.

When ROS concentrations exceed the body's scavenging abilities, O_2- reacts with NO, leading to the production of reactive nitrogen species (RNS), including peroxynitrite (ONOO–) and peroxynitrous acid (ONOOH); both compounds are highly reactive, possessing high cytotoxic activity. This process is likely the result of the phenomenon defined as "uncoupling" of the eNOS [32], which occurs following the reduction or absence of substrates, including tetrahydrobiopterin. Many conditions, including hypercholesterolemia, hypertension, and cardiovascular diseases, are commonly associated with a shortage in tetrahydrobiopterin: therefore, the resulting uncoupling of the eNOS leads to increased RNS production, reduced

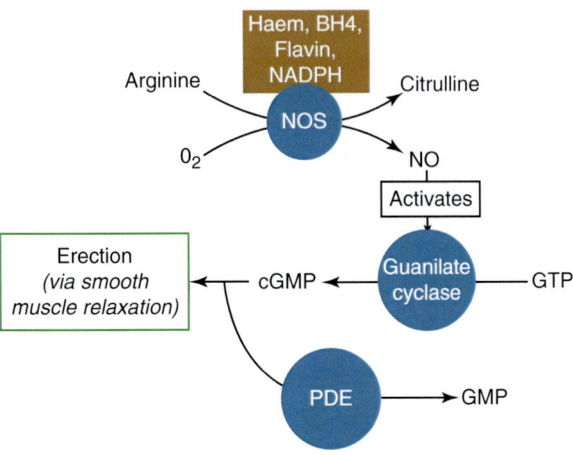

Fig. 6.1 Metabolic pathways involved in nitric oxide (NO) synthesis

NO availability, and endothelial/vascular damage. The increased production of ROS and RNS induces proliferation of smooth muscle cells and stimulates expression of ICAM-1 and VCAM-1, which in turn leads to leukocyte adhesion and migration: these mechanisms lead to oxidative stress, ultimately resulting in significant structural and functional vascular alterations [6, 45]. In the penile vascular bed, the resulting endothelial dysfunction results in impaired erectile function; therefore, administration of antioxidants has been proposed as a possible treatment for ED.

6.3.2 Antioxidant Treatment of Erectile Dysfunction

The endothelial dysfunction observed following ROS and RNS overproduction has been clearly identified as a possible cause of impaired erectile function. It is therefore unsurprising that many researchers have tried to understand whether administration of antioxidants might have an effect on ED via improvement of the NO/cGMP pathway. PDE-5 inhibitors act at the end of the pathway, by reducing the intracellular breakdown of cGMP and therefore providing longer and more valid erections; however, it has been hypothesized that administration of antioxidants might improve the scavenging systems of the penile vascular bed, thus reducing the formation of ROS and RNS.

Several different mechanisms have been investigated as possible targets for treatment [18]. As previously reported, L-arginine is a fundamental substrate for the chemical reaction leading to the formation of NO. Arginase, an enzyme competing with NOS for the substrate L-arginine, is a possible target for treatment: arginase inhibition might in fact increase the availability of serum L-arginine. In animal models, this has shown promising results both in vivo and in vitro [5, 49]; furthermore, since arginase is also involved in aberrant vessel growth and remodeling, it is possible that its inhibition might reverse or prevent vascular and endothelial dysfunction [19]. Oral administration of L-arginine does not significantly increase its serum levels because of intestinal and liver metabolism [18]; administration of L-citrulline, on the other hand, might be useful in increasing the plasmatic concentration of L-arginine. This treatment has been proven effective in rats with arterial ED [53]; in men, administration of L-carnitine has induced some improvements in men with mild forms of ED [13], with good safety and compliance profiles. Polyphenols may also act as antioxidants: resveratrol, a polyphenol commonly found in red wine, is known to improve endothelial function by activation of NOS [17] and by suppression of apoptosis [59]; similar effects have been discovered following administration of a different polyphenol, quercetin, in animal models [60].

As previously discussed, NO reacts with free radicals, ultimately resulting in production of cytotoxic compounds; antioxidants and free radical scavengers – including vitamin E, selenium, and glutathione [54] – reduce the quantity of ROS and, therefore, improve the availability of NO while at the same time reducing ROS-mediated endothelial damage [1, 10]. It has recently been hypothesized that testosterone is somehow involved in ROS production [35]: oxidative stress might be the missing link between testosterone deficiency and cardiovascular risk [56]. Literature in regard to the effects of specific antioxidant compounds in treatment of erectile function is severely lacking, despite the potential for treatment. Administration of ROS scavengers might improve the efficacy of PDE-5 inhibitors [39], as these drugs act at different levels in the NO/cGMP pathway. Oxidative stress is perhaps the common trait between some closely related conditions – cardiovascular diseases, metabolic syndrome, diabetes, lower urinary tract symptoms, and ED to name a few – which can be associated as risk factors for each other [2].

6.4 Priapism

Priapism is defined as persistent and often painful penile erection in the absence of sexual stimulation, frequently lasting more than 4 h and possibly resulting in penile fibrosis and erectile dysfunction: despite being a rare condition in the general population, its prevalence is higher among subjects with sickle cell disease or affected by perineal trauma [52]. Ischemic priapism is a medical and surgical emergency, similar to penile compartment syndrome; penile tissue shows a hypoxic and acidotic condition which requires immediate attention and might result in permanent ED if left untreated. Nonischemic priapism, occurring in about 5 % of cases, is the result of excess unregulated arterial flow to the corpora cavernosa; differently from ischemic priapism, this form is not considered an emergency, as oxygenation of the penile tissue is not interrupted. However, in almost 30 % of those affected, ED might develop despite the supposed benignity of the condition [8]: this phenomenon might be explained by the penile tissue damage associated with the traumatic development of this form of priapism.

Patients with sickle cell disease might develop a recurrent form of priapism, described as stuttering priapism, frequently occurring in their 20s; medical treatment of stuttering priapism is an emergency, although hormonal therapy for prevention of recurrences has been considered and is a viable choice [33].

6.4.1 Oxidative Stress in Priapism: A Rationale for Treatment?

Oxidative stress is increased in experimental models of priapism [29, 57], and administration of antioxidants has therefore been considered as a possible treatment for this condition. Furthermore, duration of priapism is associated with increase in oxidative stress and in antioxidant enzyme concentration [31], proving that endogenous scavenging systems might not be enough for spontaneous resolution of the condition. In animal models of ischemic priapism, some antioxidants, including pentoxifylline [12, 20], lycopene [11], and curcumin [58], have shown positive effects in reducing the oxidative damage in the cavernosal tissue. Paradoxically, enhancement of eNOS activity by a PDE-5 inhibitor (sildenafil citrate) leads to vasculoprotective effects on corpora cavernosa in rat models of stuttering priapism; by inhibiting NADPH oxidase, the chronic administration of sildenafil was able to reduce oxidative stress, once again proving that antioxidants might be helpful in treatment of specific forms of priapism [41].

Despite a growing body of evidence in support of antioxidant administration for priapism in animal models, scientific literature is lacking in regard to its viability in men. Future research should aim at identifying whether patients at risk should undergo a chronic treatment with antioxidants in order to prevent the hypoxic damage to the penile vascular bed.

> **Conclusions**
>
> As widely discussed, antioxidants are often used, albeit without solid evidence, in the treatment of several male sexual dysfunctions (Table 6.1). However, for the time being, this therapy has been suggested only as a "symptomatic" treatment. Sexual dysfunction might occur following longtime exposure to oxidative stress; therefore, identifying whether antioxidants might act as a preventive treatment for male sexual dysfunctions should be one of the most sought-after topics in future research. More and more solid evidence might suggest a potential "window of opportunity" for antioxidants in male sexual dysfunctions, resulting in a possible identification as etiological treatment.
>
> Going beyond the scope of this book, antioxidants have also been suggested as a possible therapy for female sexual dysfunctions [9]: evidence in these regards is scarce, but adequate research might provide some useful information and might help promoting antioxidants as a treatment for the benefit of the couple's sexual health.

Table 6.1 Effects of antioxidant treatment in male sexual dysfunctions

Condition	Effects of antioxidant treatment
Erectile dysfunction (ED)	Possible beneficial effects on both treatment and prevention of ED, via increased availability of nitric oxide and reduced oxidative stress
Premature ejaculation (PE)	No definite evidence of any effects, however, likely to improve conditions often associated with PE (i.e., lower urinary tract symptoms and male accessory gland infections)
Priapism	Some evidence of preventive effects in animal models; severely lacking literature in humans

References

1. Agarwal A, Nandipati KC, Sharma RK, Zippe CD, Raina R. Role of oxidative stress in the pathophysiological mechanism of erectile dysfunction. J Androl. 2006;27(3):335–47. doi:10.2164/jandrol.05136.
2. Aoun F, Albisinni S, Chemaly AK, Zanaty M, Roumeguere T. In search for a common pathway for health issues in men – the sign of a holmesian deduction. Asian Pac J Cancer Prev. 2016;17(1):1–13.
3. Atmaca M, Karadag F, Tezcan E. Serum antioxidant enzymes and malondialdehyde levels in patients with premature ejaculation before and after pharmacotherapy. J Sex Med. 2005;2(2):254–8. doi:10.1111/j.1743-6109.2005.20236.x.
4. Besiroglu H, Otunctemur A, Ozbek E. The relationship between metabolic syndrome, its components, and erectile dysfunction: a systematic review and a meta-analysis of observational studies. J Sex Med. 2015;12(6):1309–18. doi:10.1111/jsm.12885.
5. Bivalacqua TJ, Burnett AL, Hellstrom WJ, Champion HC. Overexpression of arginase in the aged mouse penis impairs erectile function and decreases eNOS activity: influence of in vivo gene therapy of anti-arginase. Am J Physiol Heart Circ Physiol. 2007;292(3):H1340–51. doi:10.1152/ajpheart.00121.2005.
6. Bryan NS, Rassaf T, Maloney RE, Rodriguez CM, Saijo F, Rodriguez JR, et al. Cellular targets and mechanisms of nitros(yl)ation: an insight into their nature and kinetics in vivo. Proc Natl Acad Sci U S A. 2004;101(12):4308–13. doi:10.1073/pnas.0306706101.
7. Burnett AL. Novel nitric oxide signaling mechanisms regulate the erectile response. Int J Impot Res. 2004;16(Suppl 1):S15–9. doi:10.1038/sj.ijir.3901209.
8. Burnett AL, Bivalacqua TJ. Priapism: new concepts in medical and surgical management. Urol Clin North Am. 2011;38(2):185–94. doi:10.1016/j.ucl.2011.02.005.
9. Caruso S, Cianci S, Cariola M, Fava V, Rapisarda A, Cianci A. Effects of nutraceuticals on quality of life and sexual function of perimenopausal women. J Endocrinol Invest. 2016; doi:10.1007/s40618-016-0500-2.
10. Castela A, Gomes P, Domingues VF, Paiga P, Costa R, Vendeira P, et al. Role of oxidative stress-induced systemic and cavernosal molecular alterations in the progression of diabetic erectile dysfunction. J Diabetes. 2015;7(3):393–401. doi:10.1111/1753-0407.12181.
11. Ciftci O, Oguz F, Beytur A, Polat F, Altintas R, Oguzturk H. Lycopene prevents experimental priapism against oxidative and nitrosative damage. Eur Rev Med Pharmacol Sci. 2014;18(21): 3320–5.
12. Cooper MA, Carrion RE, Yang C. Partial priapism treated with pentoxifylline. Int Braz J Urol. 2015;41(4):804–7. doi:10.1590/S1677-5538.IBJU.2014.0363.
13. Cormio L, De Siati M, Lorusso F, Selvaggio O, Mirabella L, Sanguedolce F, et al. Oral L-citrulline supplementation improves erection hardness in men with mild erectile dysfunction. Urology. 2011;77(1):119–22. doi:10.1016/j.urology.2010.08.028.
14. Corona G, Maggi M. Conventional and unconventional cardiovascular risk factors in men with erectile dysfunction. J Sex Med. 2013;10(2):305–8. doi:10.1111/jsm.12075.
15. Corona G, Jannini EA, Lotti F, Boddi V, De Vita G, Forti G, et al. Premature and delayed ejaculation: two ends of a single continuum influenced by hormonal milieu. Int J Androl. 2011;34(1):41–8. doi:10.1111/j.1365-2605.2010.01059.x.
16. Corona G, Gacci M, Maseroli E, Rastrelli G, Vignozzi L, Sforza A, et al. Clinical correlates of enlarged prostate size in subjects with sexual dysfunction. Asian J Androl. 2014;16(5):767–73. doi:10.4103/1008-682X.126382.
17. Dalaklioglu S, Ozbey G. The potent relaxant effect of resveratrol in rat corpus cavernosum and its underlying mechanisms. Int J Impot Res. 2013;25(5):188–93. doi:10.1038/ijir.2013.6.
18. Decaluwe K, Pauwels B, Boydens C, Van de Voorde J. Treatment of erectile dysfunction: new targets and strategies from recent research. Pharmacol Biochem Behav. 2014;121:146–57. doi:10.1016/j.pbb.2013.11.024.
19. Durante W, Johnson FK, Johnson RA. Arginase: a critical regulator of nitric oxide synthesis and vascular function. Clin Exp Pharmacol Physiol. 2007;34(9):906–11. doi:10.1111/j.1440-1681.2007.04638.x.

20. Erdemir F, Firat F, Markoc F, Atilgan D, Parlaktas BS, Kuyucu YE, et al. The effect of pentoxifylline on penile cavernosal tissues in ischemic priapism-induced rat model. Int Urol Nephrol. 2014;46(10):1961–7. doi:10.1007/s11255-014-0769-z.
21. Gazzaruso C, Coppola A, Montalcini T, Valenti C, Garzaniti A, Pelissero G, et al. Erectile dysfunction can improve the effectiveness of the current guidelines for the screening for asymptomatic coronary artery disease in diabetes. Endocrine. 2011;40(2):273–9. doi:10.1007/s12020-011-9523-9.
22. Ghanem HM, Salonia A, Martin-Morales A. SOP: physical examination and laboratory testing for men with erectile dysfunction. J Sex Med. 2013;10(1):108–10. doi:10.1111/j.1743-6109.2012.02734.x.
23. Iii Colado-Velazquez J, Mailloux-Salinas P, Medina-Contreras J, Cruz-Robles D, Bravo G. Effect of Serenoa Repens on oxidative stress, inflammatory and growth factors in obese wistar rats with benign prostatic hyperplasia. Phytother Res. 2015;29(10):1525–31. doi:10.1002/ptr.5406.
24. Jannini EA, Lenzi A. Epidemiology of premature ejaculation. Curr Opin Urol. 2005;15(6):399–403.
25. Jannini EA, Lombardo F, Lenzi A. Correlation between ejaculatory and erectile dysfunction. Int J Androl. 2005;28(Suppl 2):40–5. doi:10.1111/j.1365-2605.2005.00593.x.
26. Jannini EA, Lenzi A, Isidori A, Fabbri A. Subclinical erectile dysfunction: proposal for a novel taxonomic category in sexual medicine. J Sex Med 2006;3(5):787–93. doi:10.1111/j.1743--6109.2006.00287.x; discussion 94.
27. Jannini EA, McCabe MP, Salonia A, Montorsi F, Sachs BD. Organic vs. psychogenic? The Manichean diagnosis in sexual medicine. J Sex Med. 2010;7(5):1726–33. doi:10.1111/j.1743-6109.2010.01824.x.
28. Jannini EA, Isidori AM, Aversa A, Lenzi A, Althof SE. Which is first? The controversial issue of precedence in the treatment of male sexual dysfunctions. J Sex Med. 2013;10(10):2359–69. doi:10.1111/jsm.12315.
29. Kanika ND, Melman A, Davies KP. Experimental priapism is associated with increased oxidative stress and activation of protein degradation pathways in corporal tissue. Int J Impot Res. 2010;22(6):363–73. doi:10.1038/ijir.2010.27.
30. Kaya E, Sikka SC, Gur S. A comprehensive review of metabolic syndrome affecting erectile dysfunction. J Sex Med. 2015;12(4):856–75. doi:10.1111/jsm.12828.
31. Kucukdurmaz F, Kucukgergin C, Akman T, Salabas E, Armagan A, Seckin S, et al. Duration of priapism is associated with increased corporal oxidative stress and antioxidant enzymes in a rat model. Andrologia. 2016;48(4):374–9. doi:10.1111/and.12455.
32. Landmesser U, Dikalov S, Price SR, McCann L, Fukai T, Holland SM, et al. Oxidation of tetrahydrobiopterin leads to uncoupling of endothelial cell nitric oxide synthase in hypertension. J Clin Invest. 2003;111(8):1201–9. doi:10.1172/JCI14172.
33. Levey HR, Segal RL, Bivalacqua TJ. Management of priapism: an update for clinicians. Ther Adv Urol. 2014;6(6):230–44. doi:10.1177/1756287214542096.
34. Lewis RW, Fugl-Meyer KS, Corona G, Hayes RD, Laumann EO, Moreira Jr ED, et al. Definitions/epidemiology/risk factors for sexual dysfunction. J Sex Med. 2010;7(4 Pt 2):1598–607. doi:10.1111/j.1743-6109.2010.01778.x.
35. Li R, Meng X, Zhang Y, Wang T, Yang J, Niu Y, et al. Testosterone improves erectile function through inhibition of reactive oxygen species generation in castrated rats. Peer J. 2016;4:e2000. doi:10.7717/peerj.2000.
36. Limoncin E, Tomassetti M, Gravina GL, Ciocca G, Carosa E, Di Sante S, et al. Premature ejaculation results in female sexual distress: standardization and validation of a new diagnostic tool for sexual distress. J Urol. 2013;189(5):1830–5. doi:10.1016/j.juro.2012.11.007.
37. McCarty EJ, Dinsmore WW. Premature ejaculation: treatment update. Int J STD AIDS. 2010;21(2):77–81. doi:10.1258/ijsa.2009.009434.
38. McMahon CG, Jannini E, Waldinger M, Rowland D. Standard operating procedures in the disorders of orgasm and ejaculation. J Sex Med. 2013;10(1):204–29. doi:10.1111/j.1743-6109.2012.02824.x.
39. Meldrum DR, Burnett AL, Dorey G, Esposito K, Ignarro LJ. Erectile hydraulics: maximizing inflow while minimizing outflow. J Sex Med. 2014;11(5):1208–20. doi:10.1111/jsm.12457.

40. Musicki B, Ross AE, Champion HC, Burnett AL, Bivalacqua TJ. Posttranslational modification of constitutive nitric oxide synthase in the penis. J Androl. 2009;30(4):352–62. doi:10.2164/jandrol.108.006999.
41. Musicki B, Bivalacqua TJ, Champion HC, Burnett AL. Sildenafil promotes eNOS activation and inhibits NADPH oxidase in the transgenic sickle cell mouse penis. J Sex Med. 2014;11(2):424–30. doi:10.1111/jsm.12391.
42. NIH Consensus Conference Impotence. NIH consensus development panel on impotence. JAMA. 1993;270(1):83–90.
43. Omu AE, Al-Bader AA, Dashti H, Oriowo MA. Magnesium in human semen: possible role in premature ejaculation. Arch Androl. 2001;46(1):59–66.
44. Otunctemur A, Ozbek E, Kirecci SL, Ozcan L, Dursun M, Cekmen M, et al. Relevance of serum nitric oxide levels and the efficacy of selective serotonin reuptake inhibitors treatment on premature ejaculation: decreased nitric oxide is associated with premature ejaculation. Andrologia. 2014;46(9):951–5. doi:10.1111/and.12179.
45. Pierini D, Bryan NS. Nitric oxide availability as a marker of oxidative stress. Methods Mol Biol. 2015;1208:63–71. doi:10.1007/978-1-4939-1441-8_5.
46. Romanelli F, Sansone A, Lenzi A. Erectile dysfunction in aging male. Acta Biomed. 2010;81(Suppl 1):89–94.
47. Sansone A, Romanelli F, Gianfrilli D, Lenzi A. Endocrine evaluation of erectile dysfunction. Endocrine. 2014;46(3):423–30. doi:10.1007/s12020-014-0254-6.
48. Sansone A, Romanelli F, Jannini EA, Lenzi A. Hormonal correlations of premature ejaculation. Endocrine. 2015;49(2):333–8. doi:10.1007/s12020-014-0520-7.
49. Segal R, Hannan JL, Liu X, Kutlu O, Burnett AL, Champion HC, et al. Chronic oral administration of the arginase inhibitor 2(S)-amino-6-boronohexanoic acid (ABH) improves erectile function in aged rats. J Androl. 2012;33(6):1169–75. doi:10.2164/jandrol.111.015834.
50. Selvin E, Burnett AL, Platz EA. Prevalence and risk factors for erectile dysfunction in the US. Am J Med. 2007;120(2):151–7. doi:10.1016/j.amjmed.2006.06.010.
51. Shamloul R, Ghanem H. Erectile dysfunction. Lancet. 2013;381(9861):153–65. doi:10.1016/S0140-6736(12)60520-0.
52. Shigehara K, Namiki M. Clinical management of priapism: a review. World J Mens Health. 2016;34(1):1–8. doi:10.5534/wjmh.2016.34.1.1.
53. Shiota A, Hotta Y, Kataoka T, Morita M, Maeda Y, Kimura K. Oral L-citrulline supplementation improves erectile function in rats with acute arteriogenic erectile dysfunction. J Sex Med. 2013;10(10):2423–9. doi:10.1111/jsm.12260.
54. Tagliabue M, Pinach S, Di Bisceglie C, Brocato L, Cassader M, Bertagna A, et al. Glutathione levels in patients with erectile dysfunction, with or without diabetes mellitus. Int J Androl. 2005;28(3):156–62. doi:10.1111/j.1365-2605.2005.00528.x.
55. Teles AG, Carreira M, Alarcao V, Sociol D, Aragues JM, Lopes L, et al. Prevalence, severity, and risk factors for erectile dysfunction in a representative sample of 3,548 portuguese men aged 40 to 69 years attending primary healthcare centers: results of the Portuguese erectile dysfunction study. J Sex Med. 2008;5(6):1317–24. doi:10.1111/j.1743-6109.2007.00745.x.
56. Tostes RC, Carneiro FS, Carvalho MH, Reckelhoff JF. Reactive oxygen species: players in the cardiovascular effects of testosterone. Am J Physiol Regul Integr Comp Physiol. 2016;310(1):R1–14. doi:10.1152/ajpregu.00392.2014.
57. Wood KC, Hsu LL, Gladwin MT. Sickle cell disease vasculopathy: a state of nitric oxide resistance. Free Radic Biol Med. 2008;44(8):1506–28. doi:10.1016/j.freeradbiomed.2008.01.008.
58. Yilmaz Y, Taken K, Atar M, Ergun M, Soylemez H. Protective effect of curcumin on priapism and ischemia-reperfusion injury in rats. Eur Rev Med Pharmacol Sci. 2015;19(23):4664–70.
59. Yu W, Wan Z, Qiu XF, Chen Y, Dai YT. Resveratrol, an activator of SIRT1, restores erectile function in streptozotocin-induced diabetic rats. Asian J Androl. 2013;15(5):646–51. doi:10.1038/aja.2013.60.
60. Zhang W, Wang Y, Yang Z, Qiu J, Ma J, Zhao Z, et al. Antioxidant treatment with quercetin ameliorates erectile dysfunction in streptozotocin-induced diabetic rats. J Biosci Bioeng. 2011;112(3):215–8. doi:10.1016/j.jbiosc.2011.05.013.

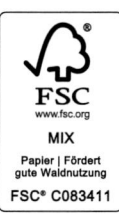

FSC
www.fsc.org
MIX
Papier | Fördert
gute Waldnutzung
FSC® C083411

Zeitfracht Medien GmbH
Ferdinand-Jühlke-Straße 7
99095 Erfurt, Deutschland
produktsicherheit@kolibri360.de